CAPTAIN CHEMO!

Childhood Illness

Book 1

RENEE ROBINSON

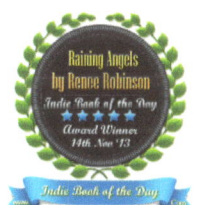

DEDICATION

To the children who fight to live. To the children who fought and won. To the children who will fight in the future. Hold onto Captain Chemo and be strong just like him. Think of happy thoughts when you are down and remember hope never runs out.

CONTENTS

ACKNOWLEDGMENTS

Images © 2013 GraphicFactory
Image © Graphics Factory.com

Illustrations: Graphics Factory.com memberships include a royalty-free license to use any of the 2,367,983 images for commercial projects. Your license to use any of the 2.3 Million plus images in accordance with the Graphics Factory terms. It really doesn't get any easier or more affordable to use images for your products for almost any purpose: commercial, educational or personal.

Images: © 2014 free-graphics.com
Additional Images & Illustrations are the product of: http://www.iCLIPART.com - 7.8 Million Images. www.free-graphics.com & http://www.thefreesite.com/

1 Captain Chemo

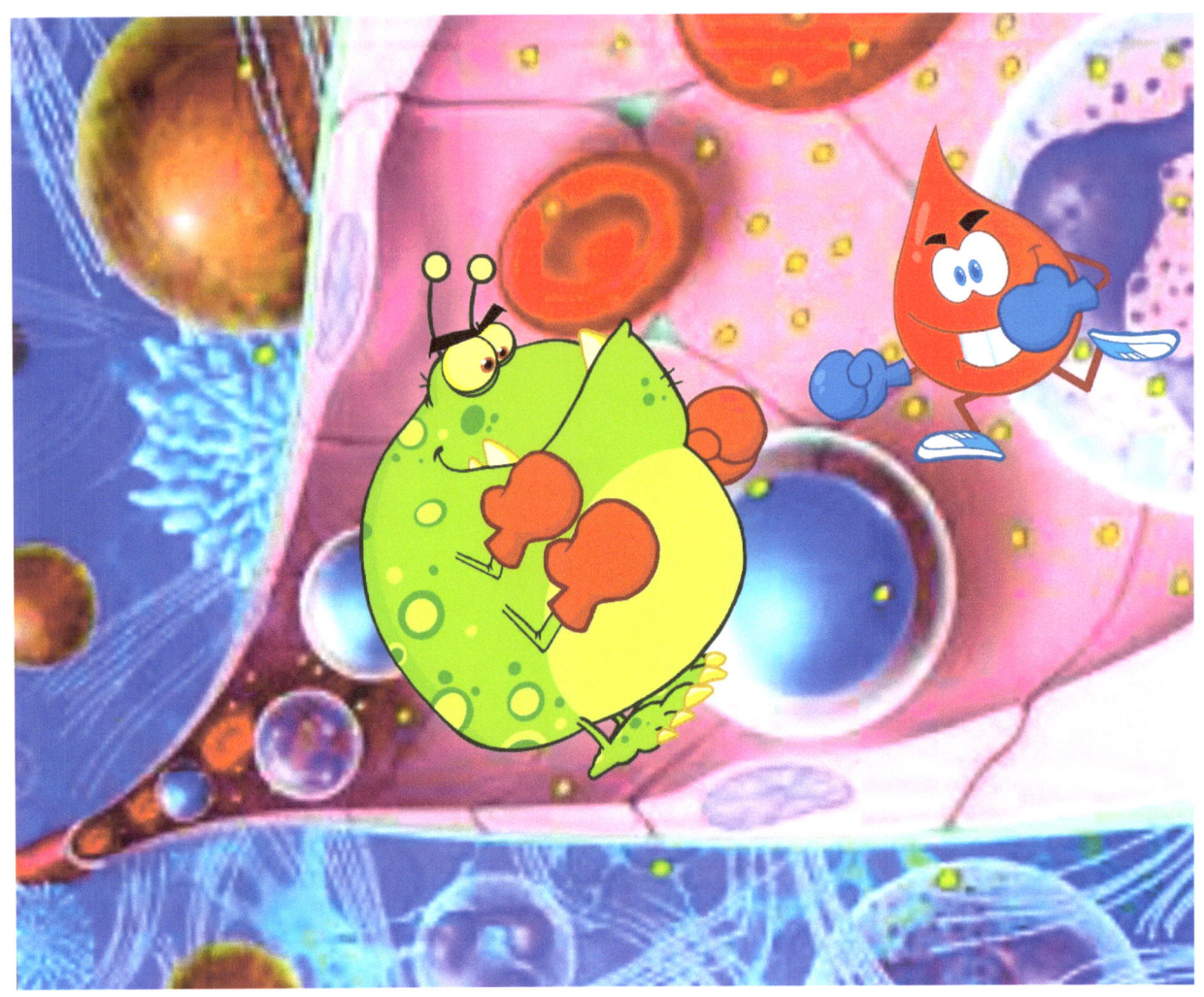

Out Cancer, out! Do you hear me?
This body is mine! Not yours and your family's.

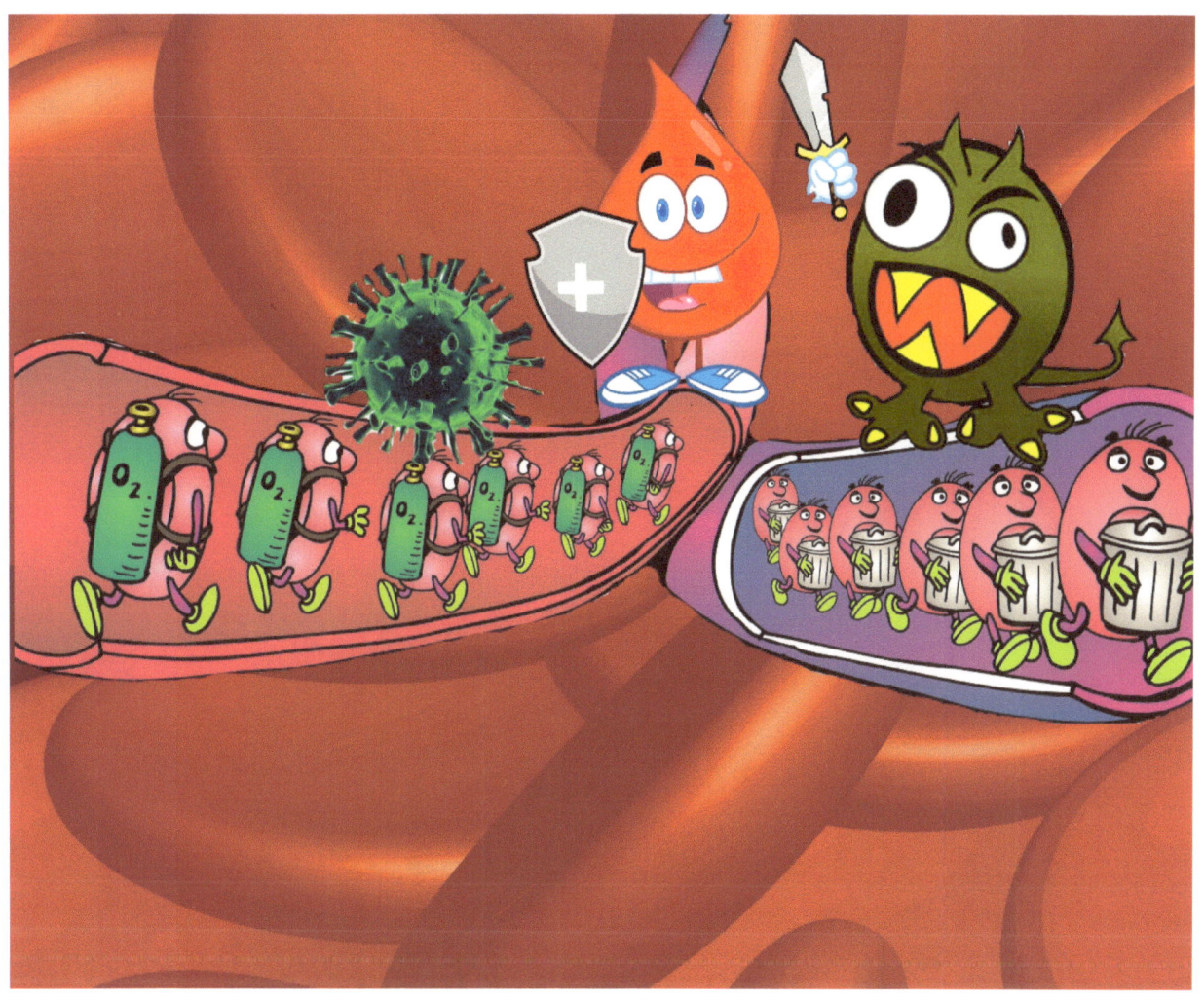

You are a mutated cell swimming in my bloodstream.

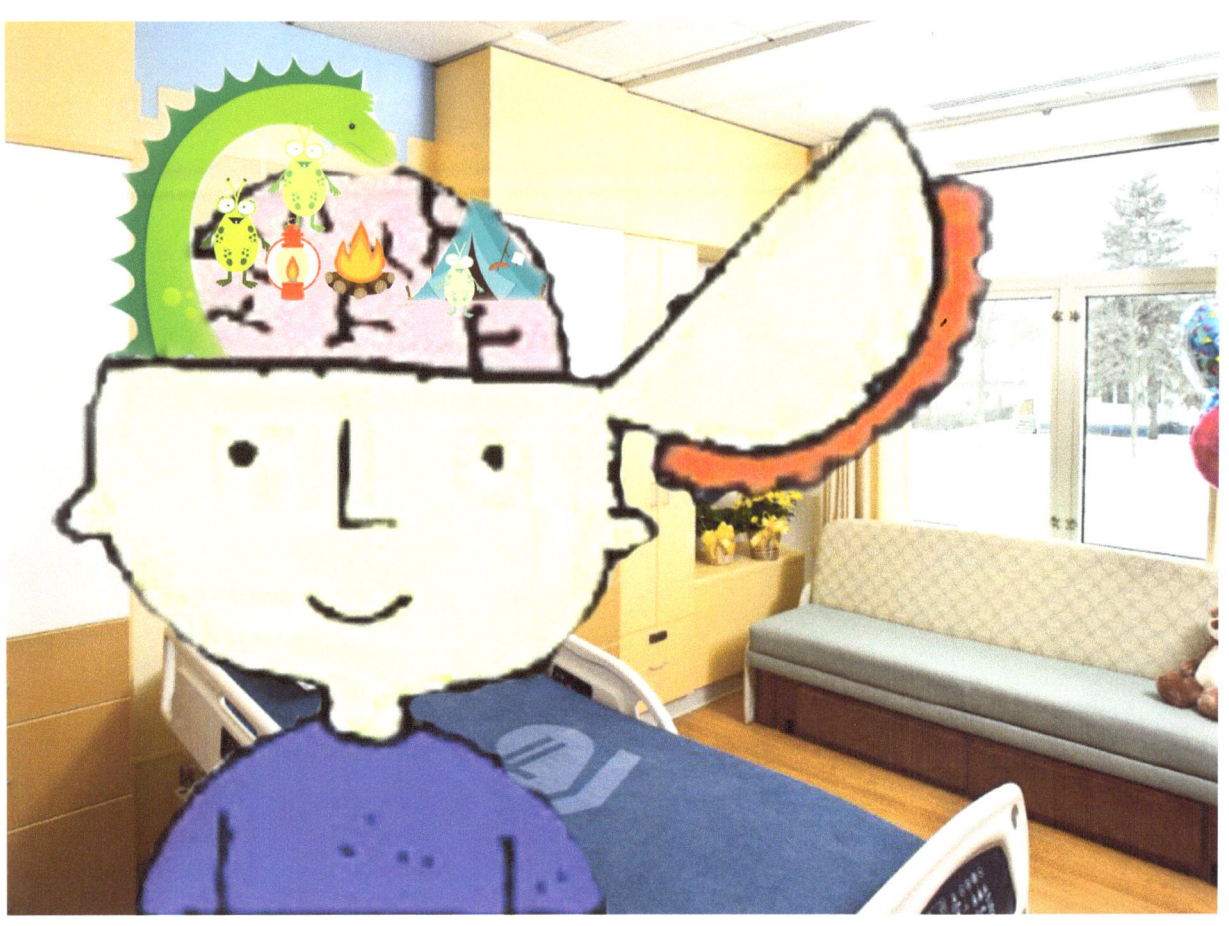

Looking for a place to stay
for you and your Mutant Team

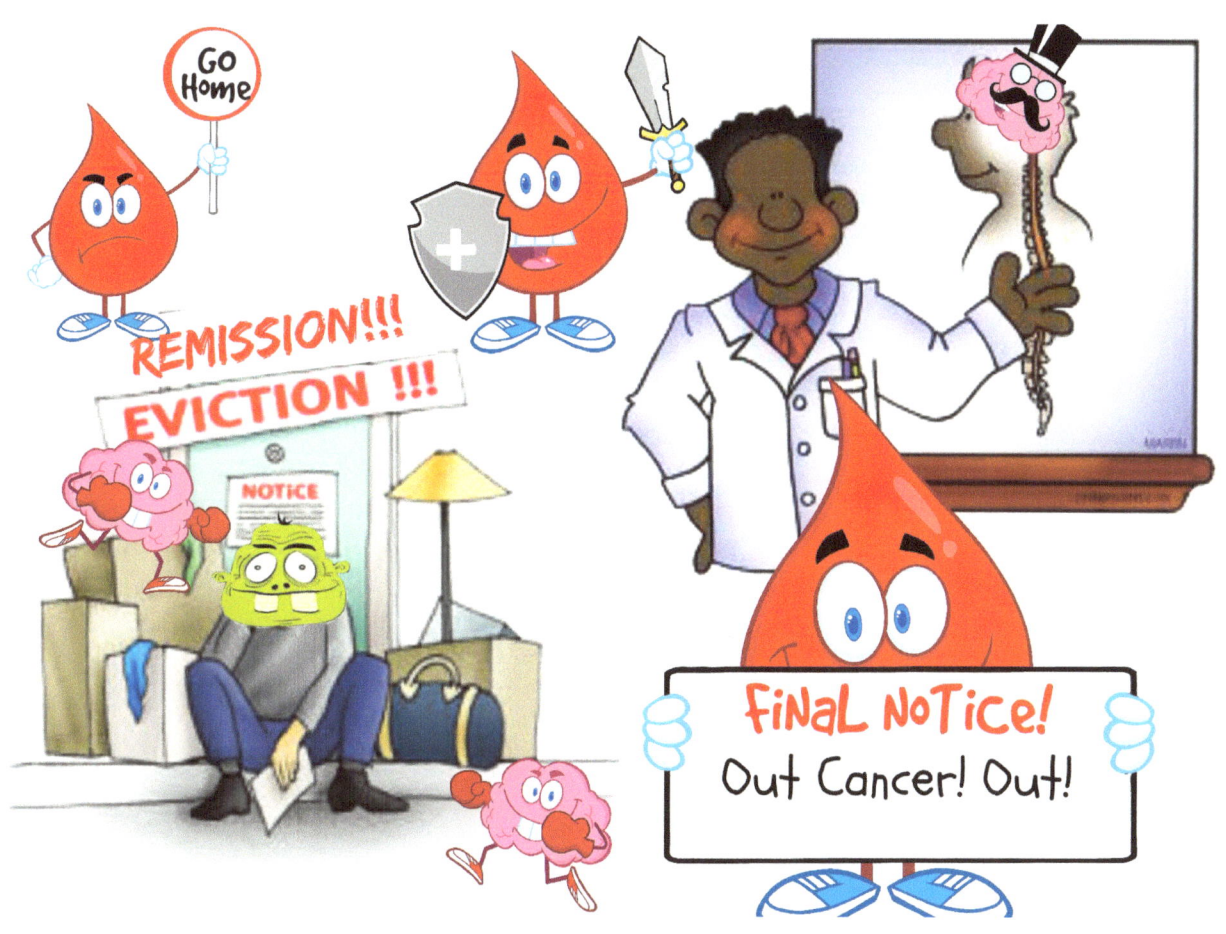

I have a friend named Captain Chemo.
He is here to toss you out.
You will be evicted.
Out Cancer, out!

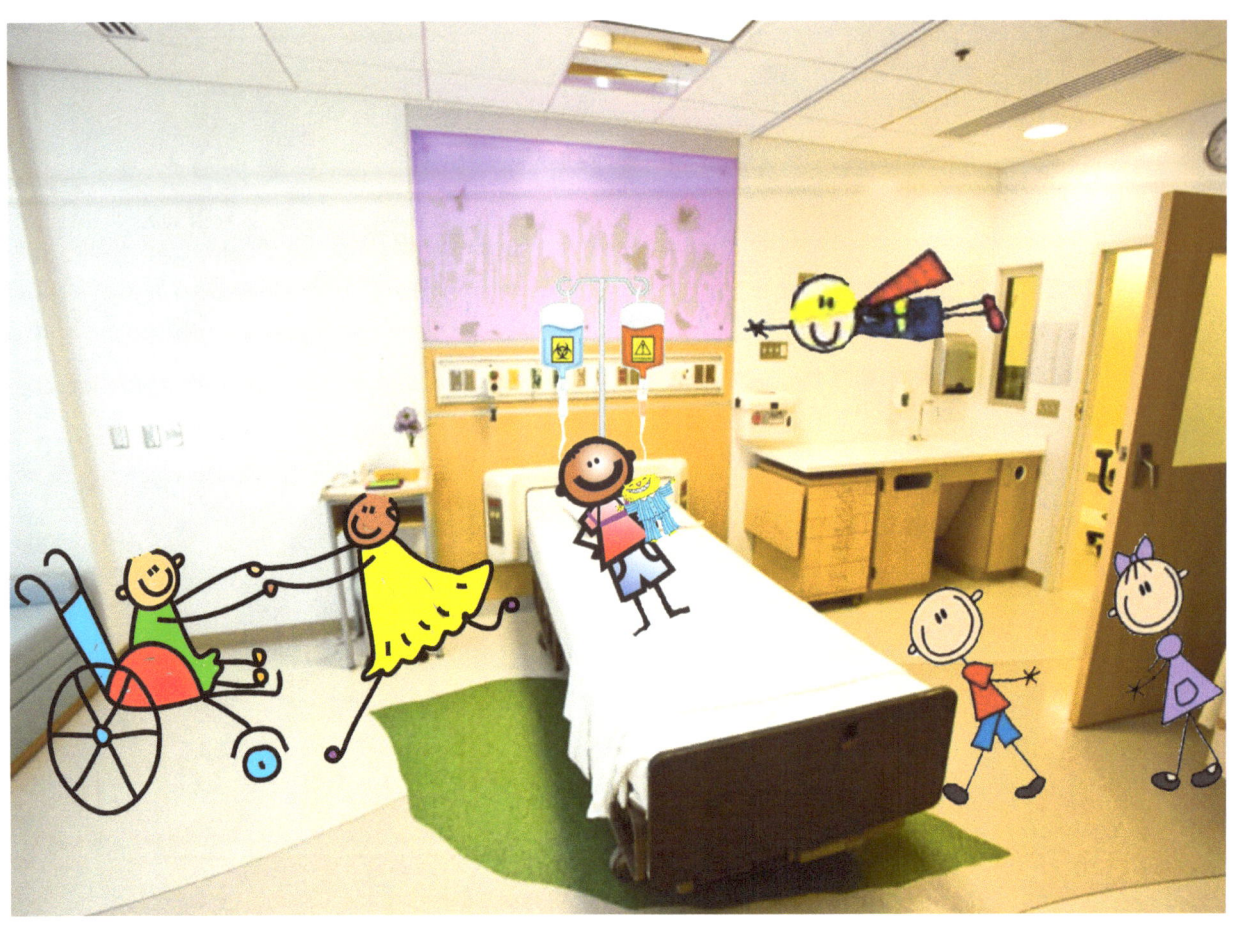

I may lose all of my hair
But I hope to win life

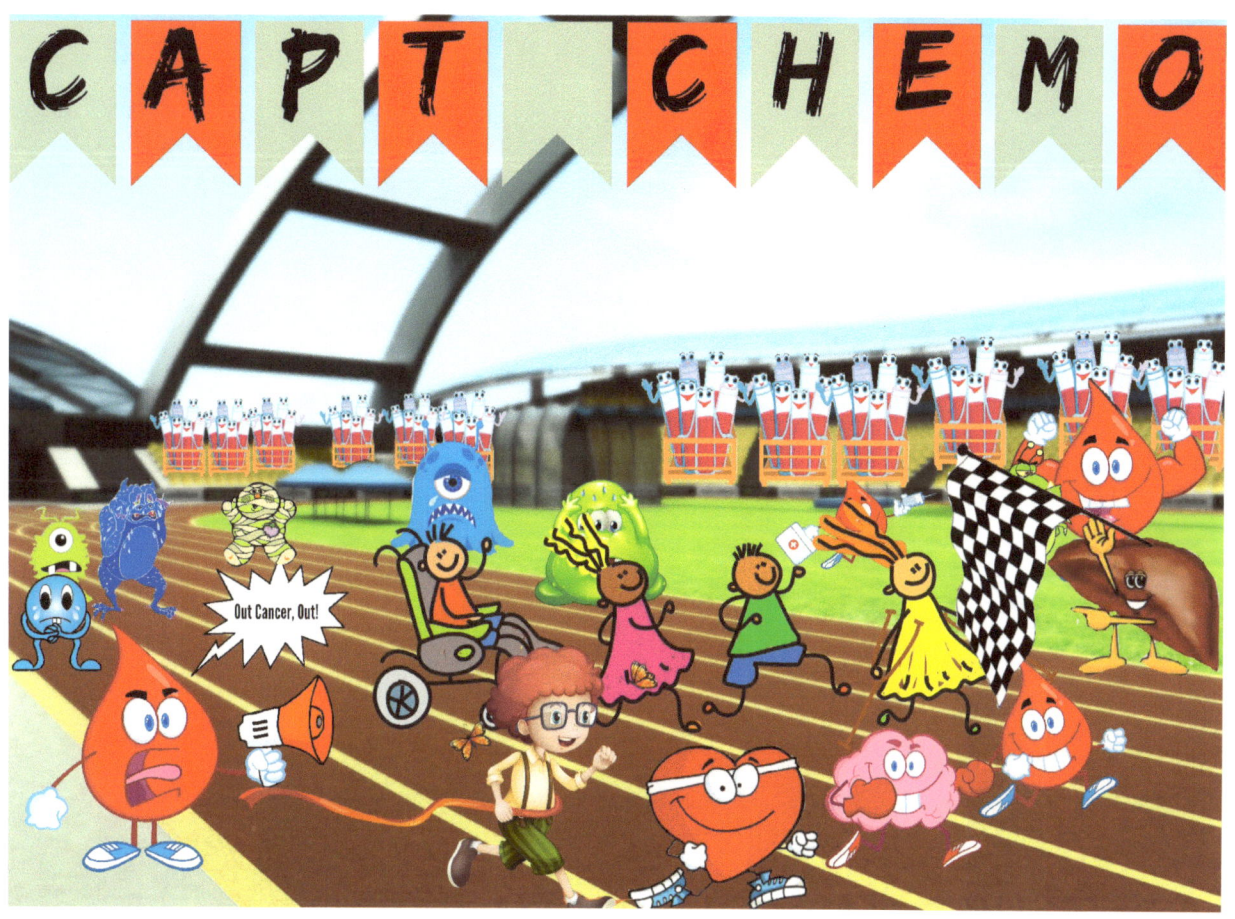

Cancer will be beaten
Captain Chemo is on my side

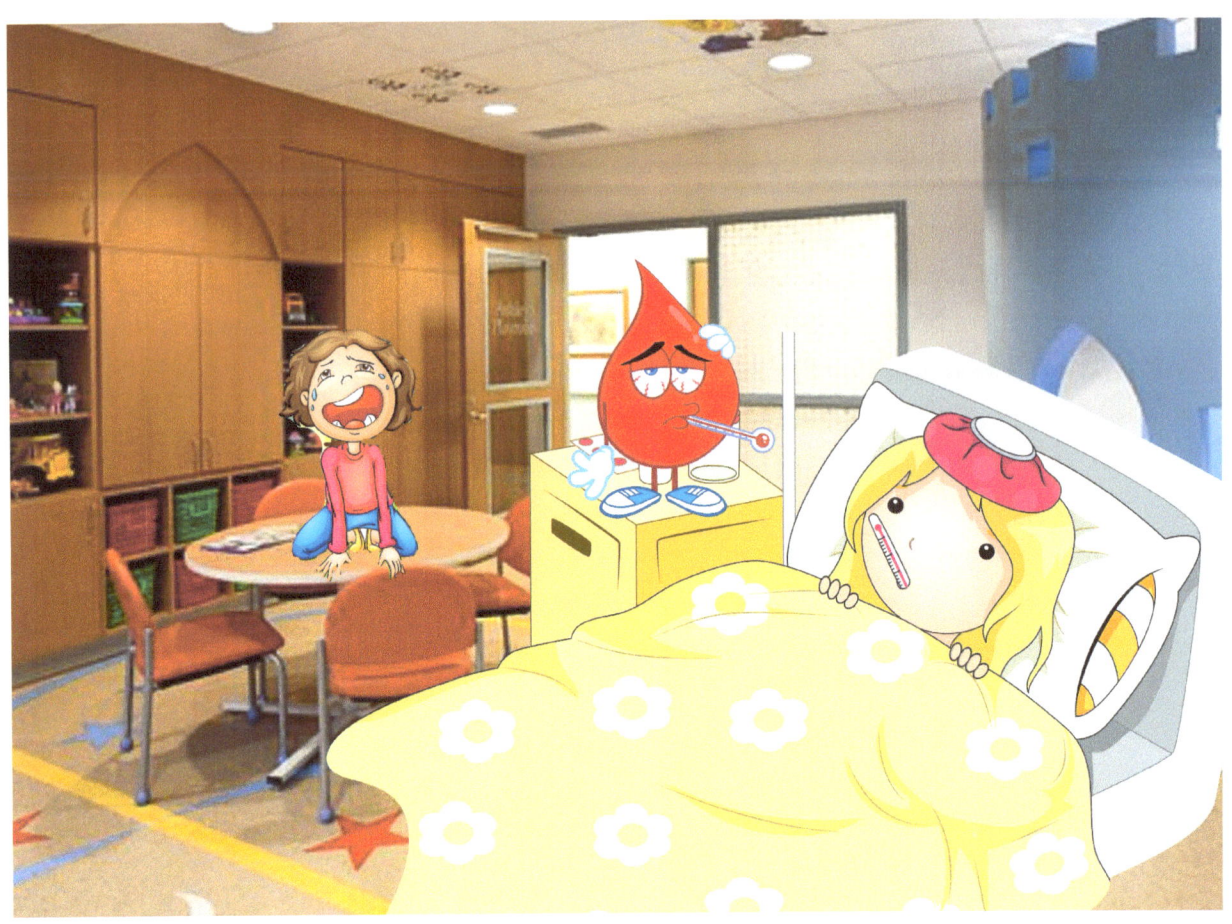

Your pain makes me cry
It makes me very sad

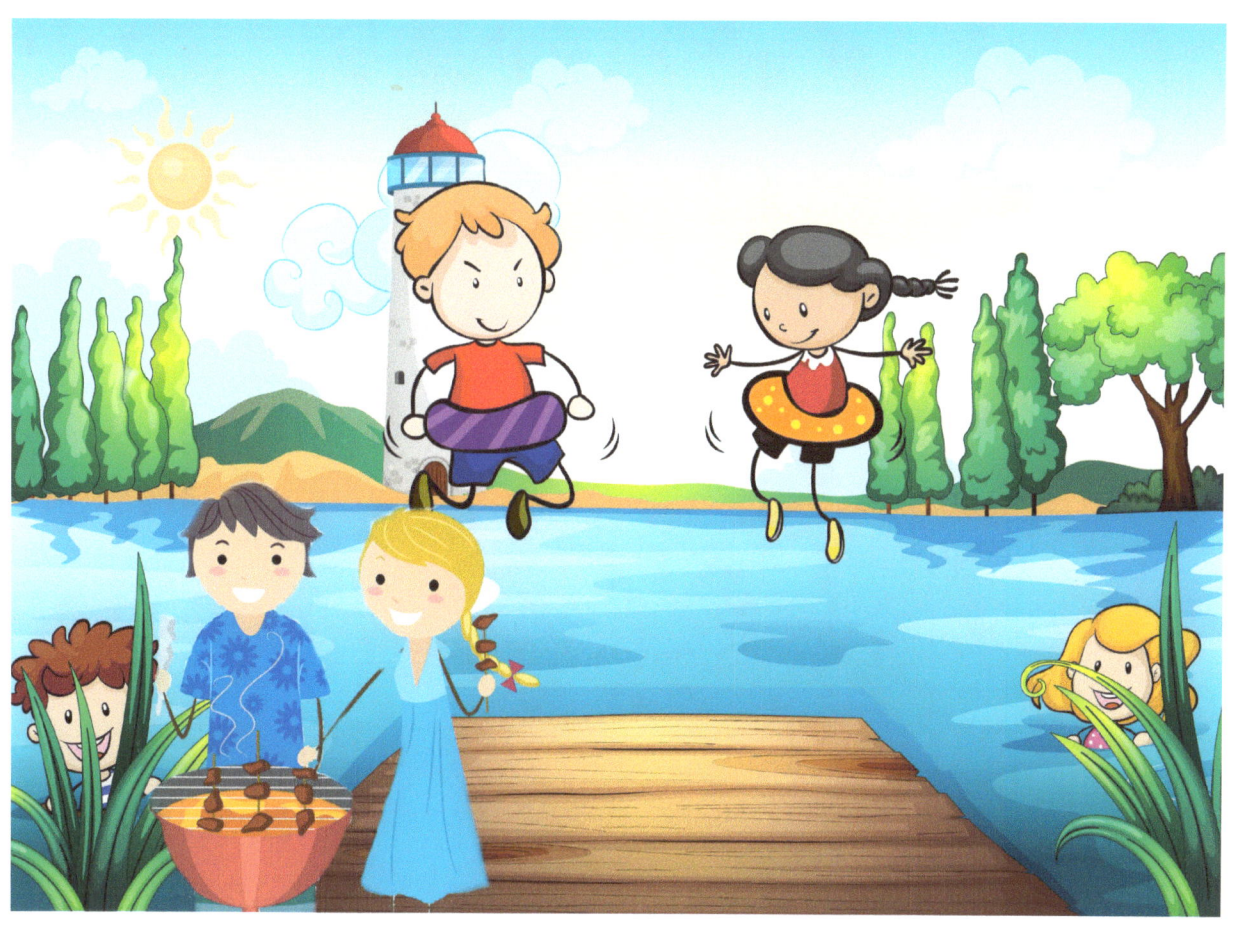

So I think of happy times
Like playing with my dad

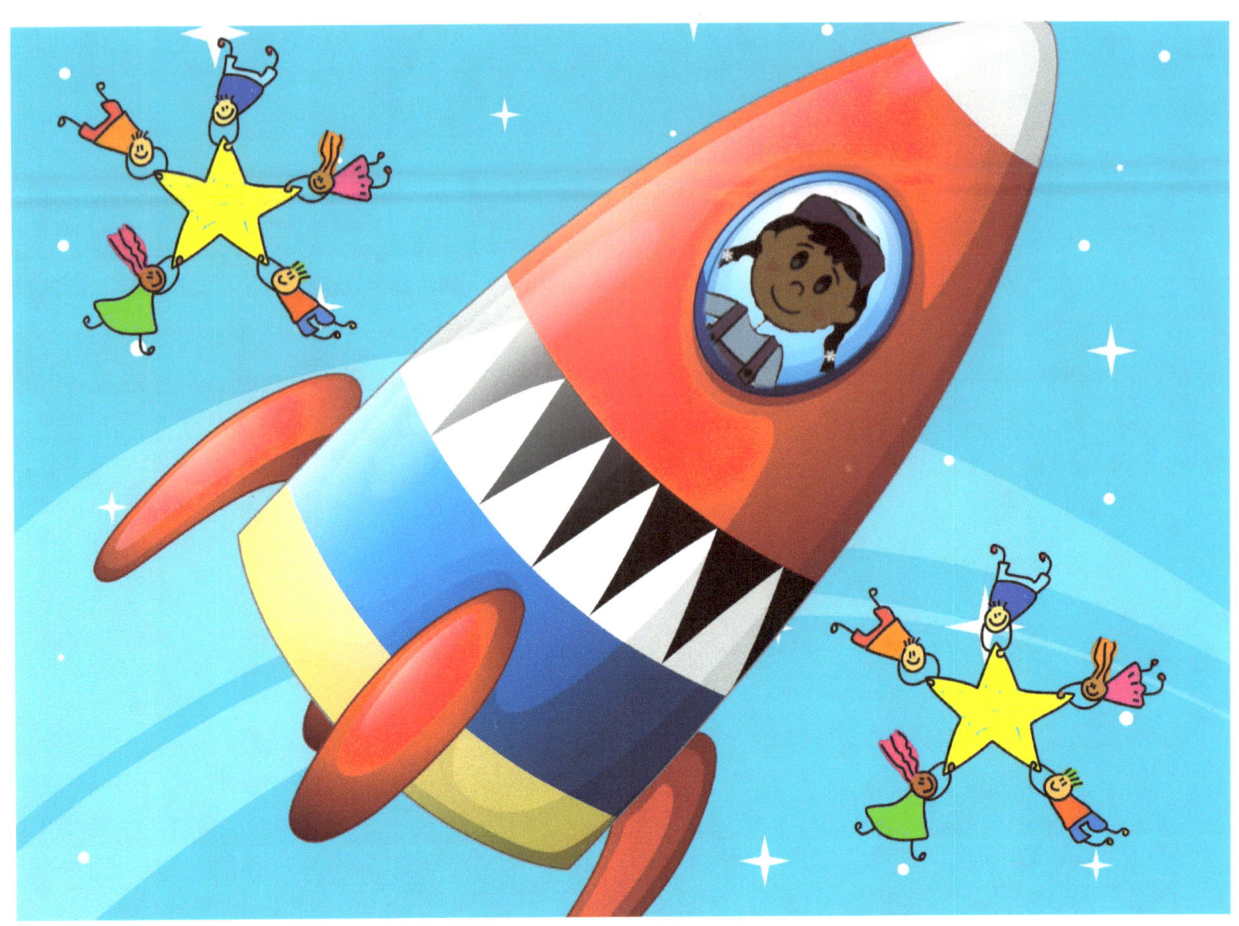

I will dream of a spaceship
And catching a star

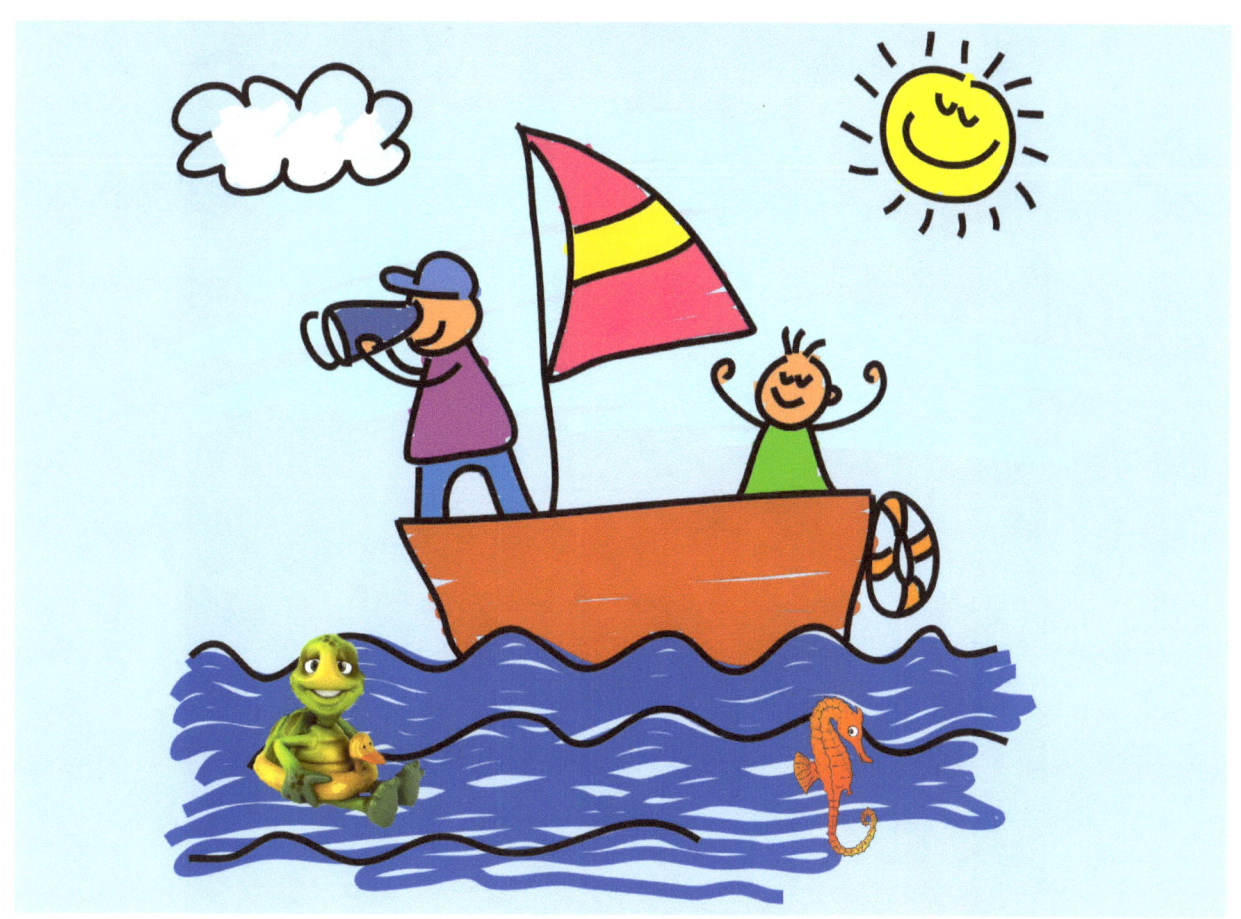

Or I will sail on a great ship
I will travel afar

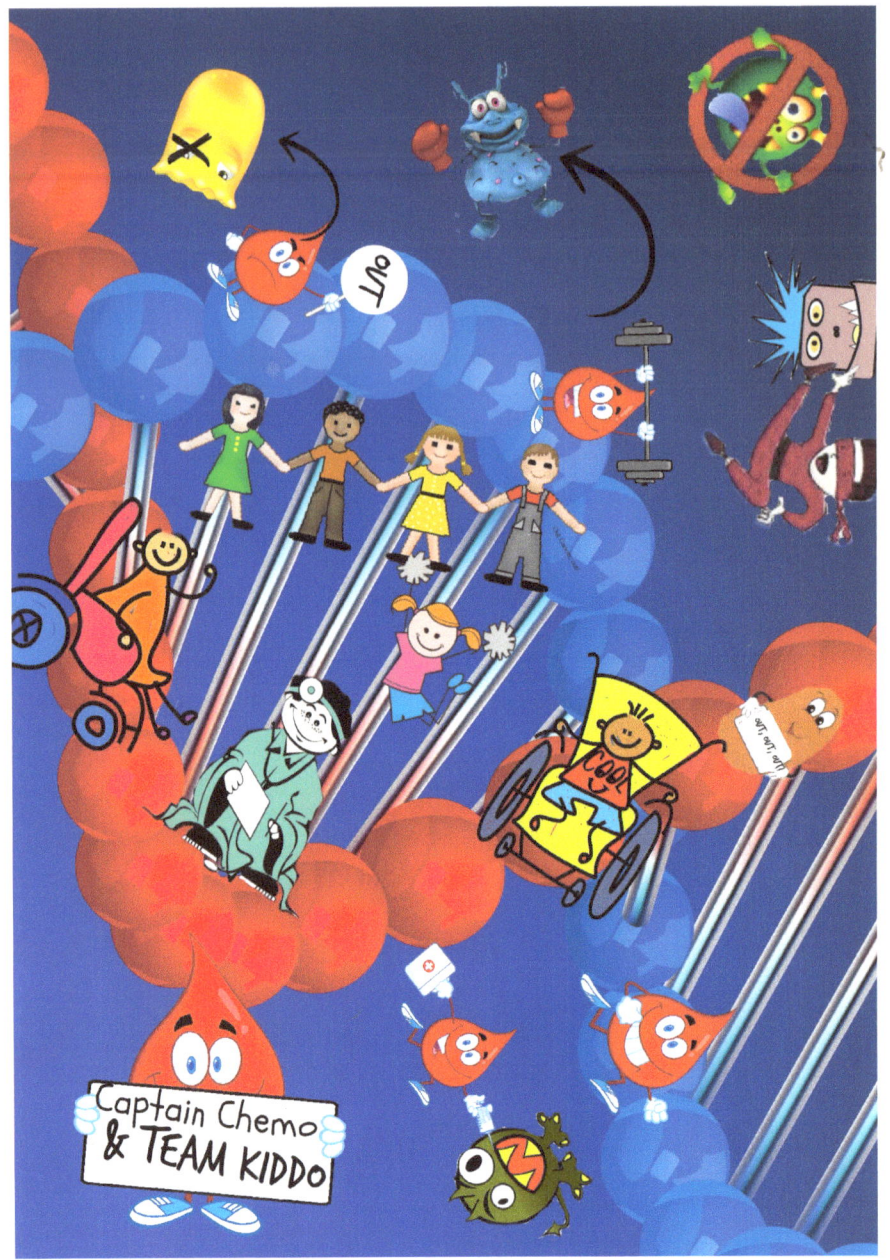

Captain Chemo will come again
Together we continue to fight

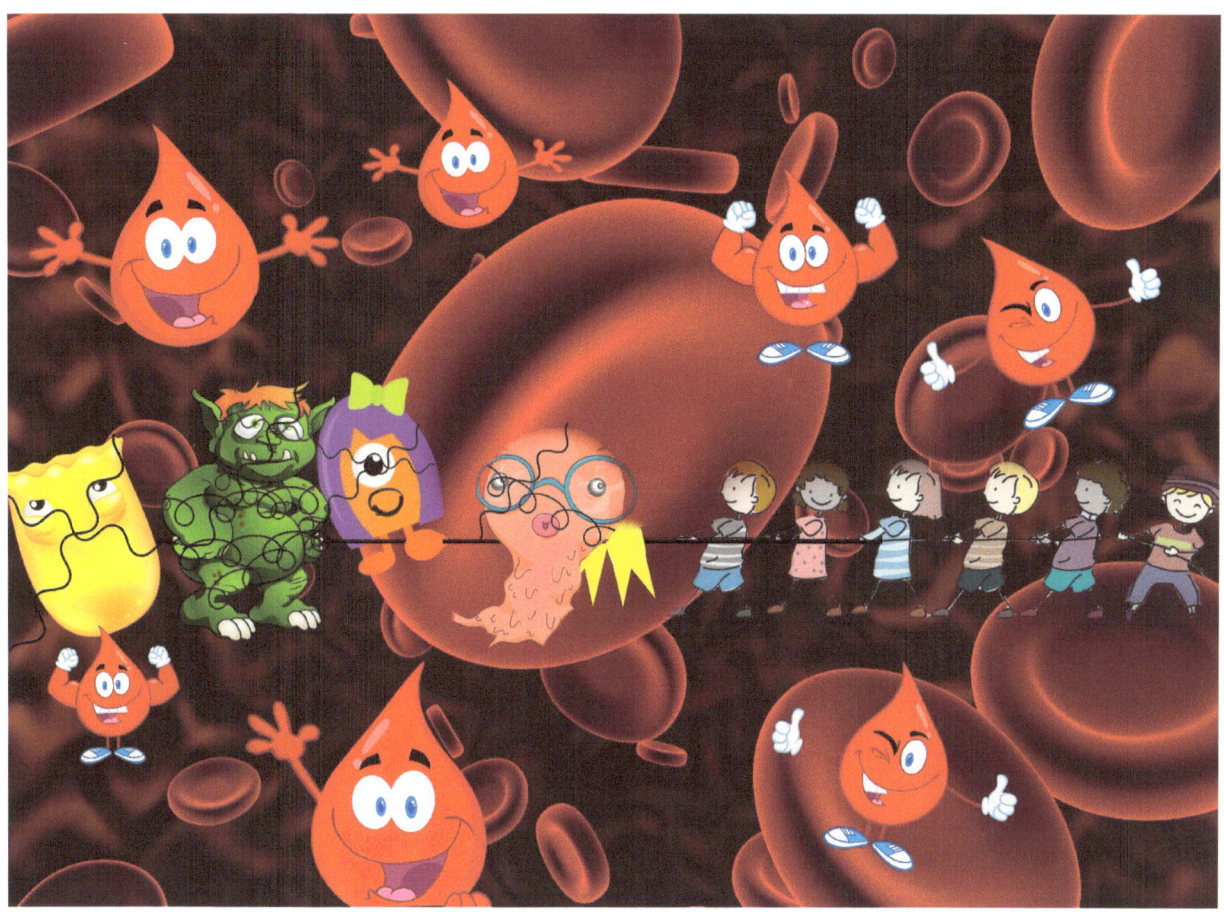

It is a long hard war
It seems no end is in sight

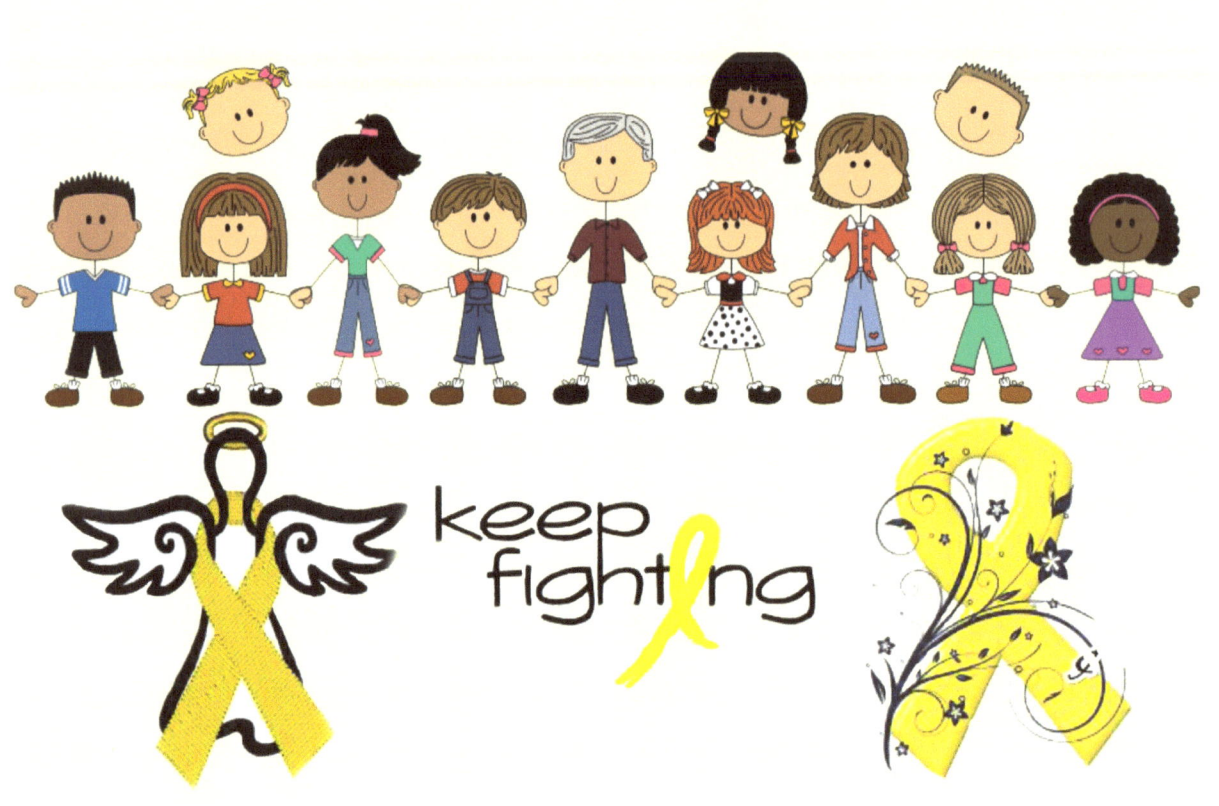

But I have Love and Hope on my side
Within my family and friends

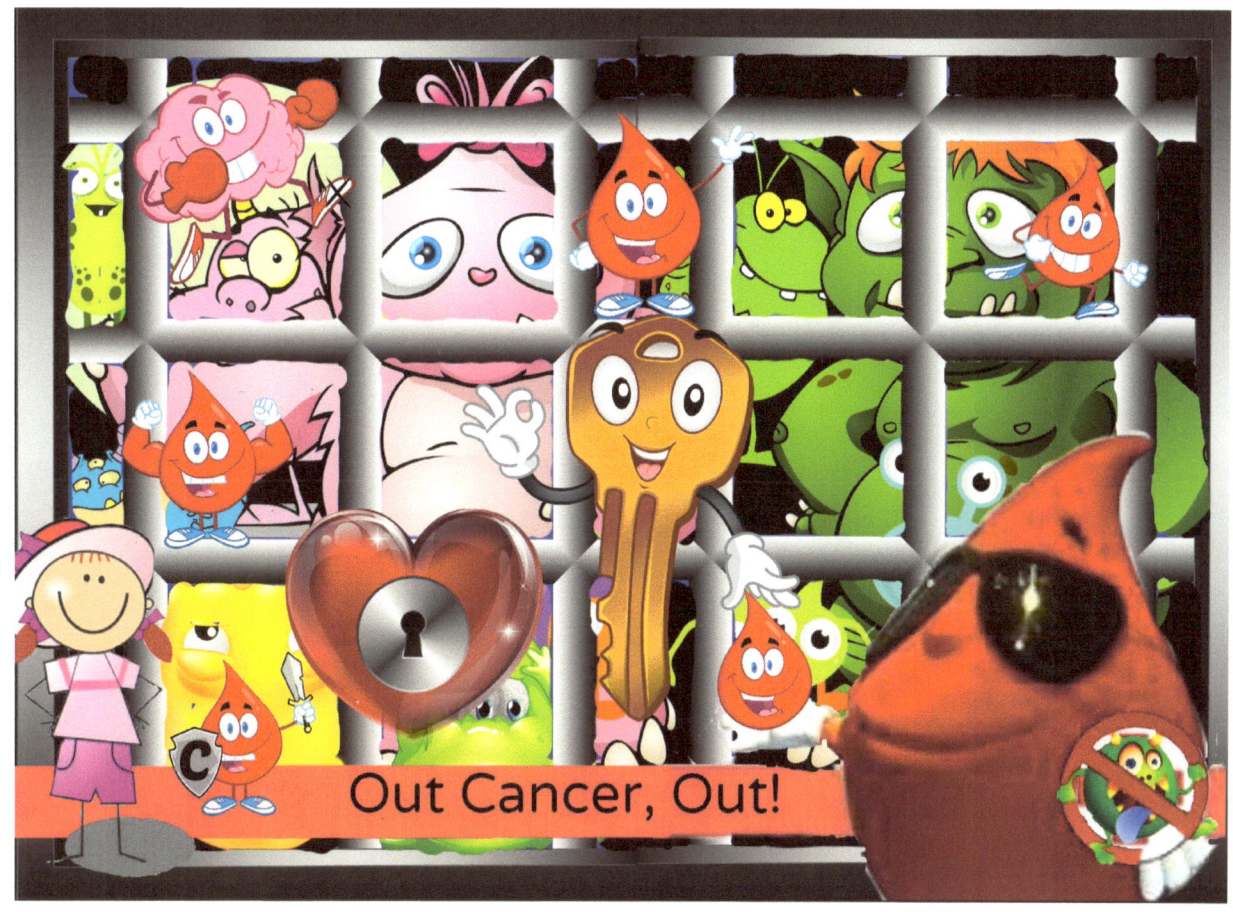

We are bigger and stronger
We will fight to the end

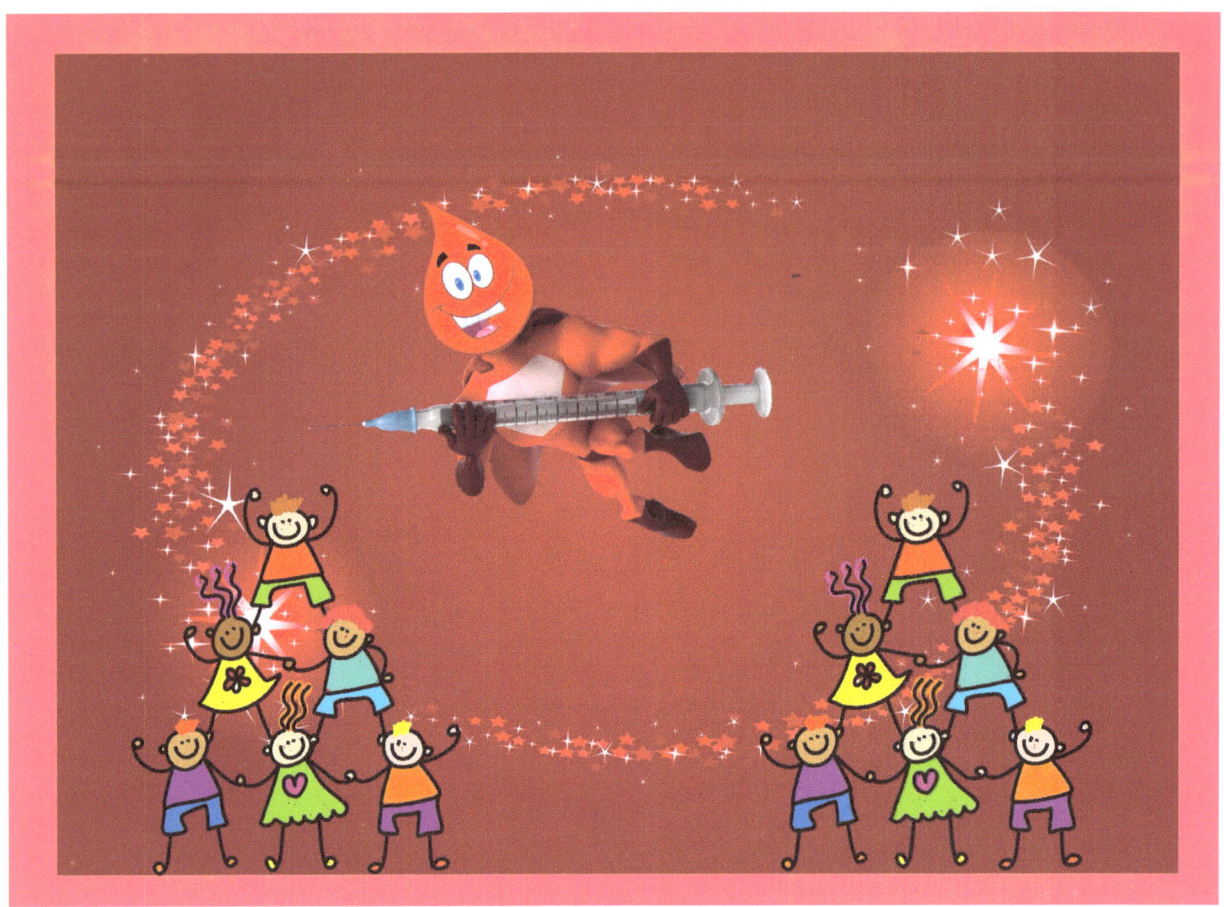

And Captain Chemo is still here too
He is going to toss you out.
You will be evicted.
Out Cancer, out!

2 COLOR THE CHARACTERS

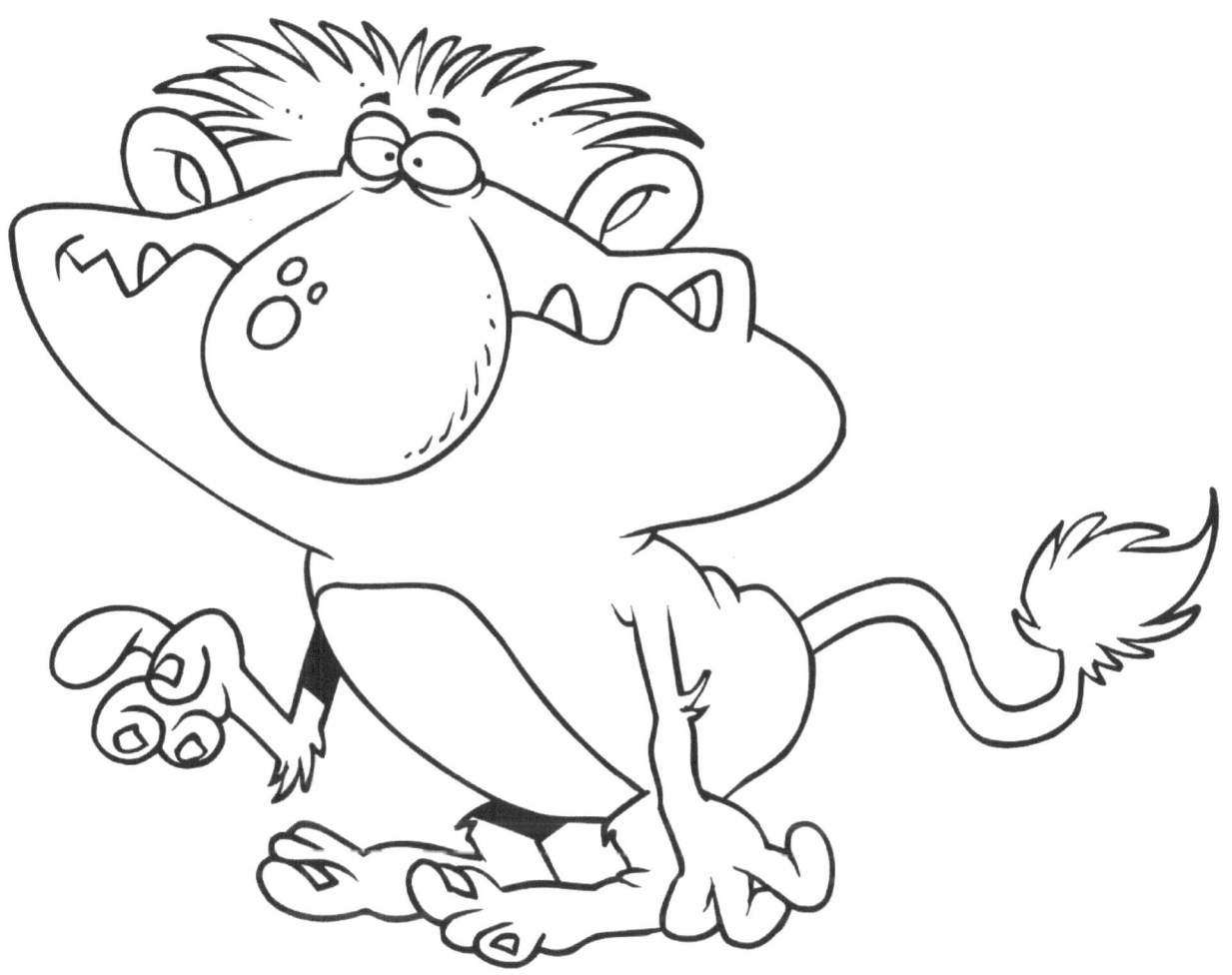

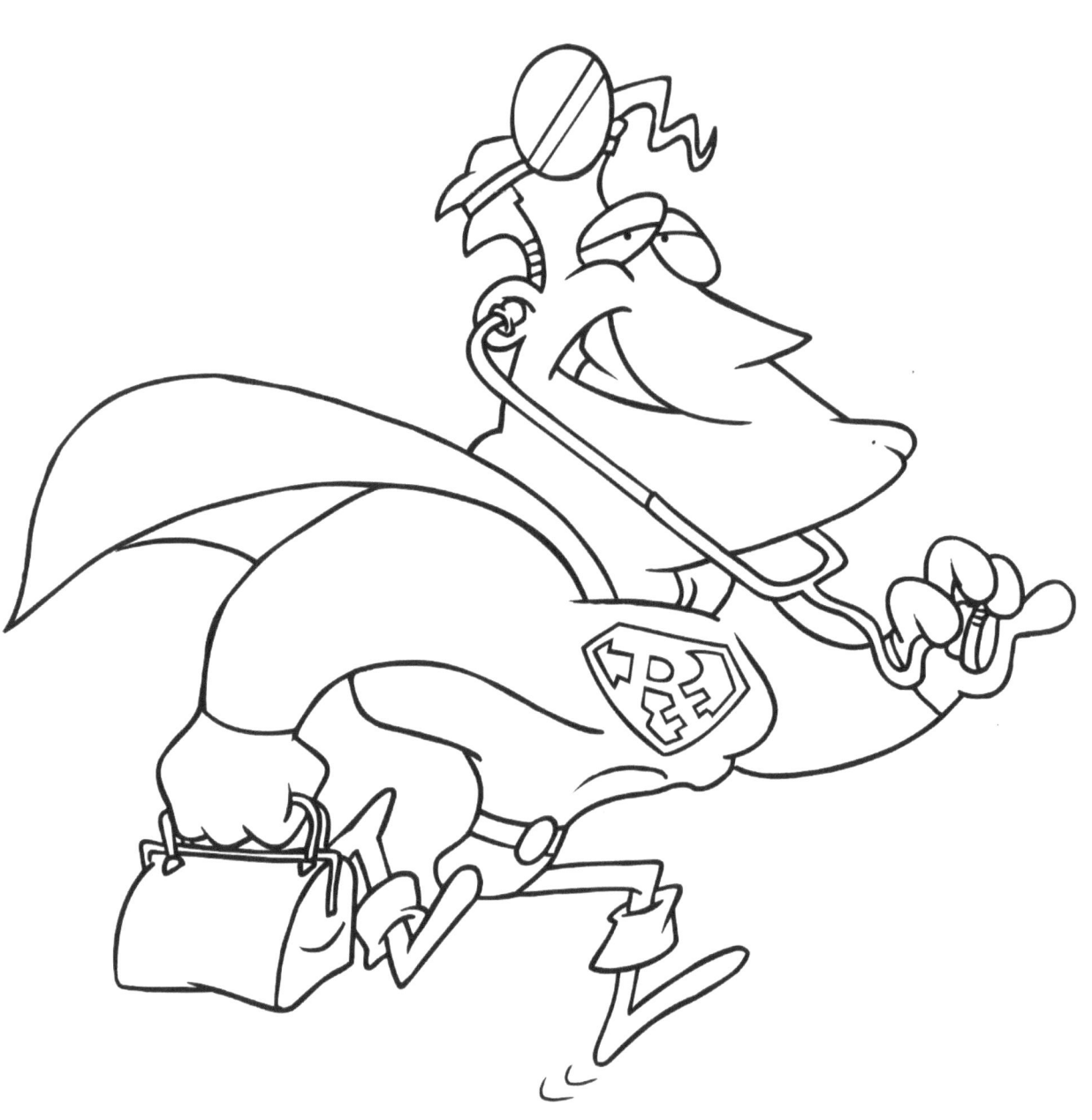

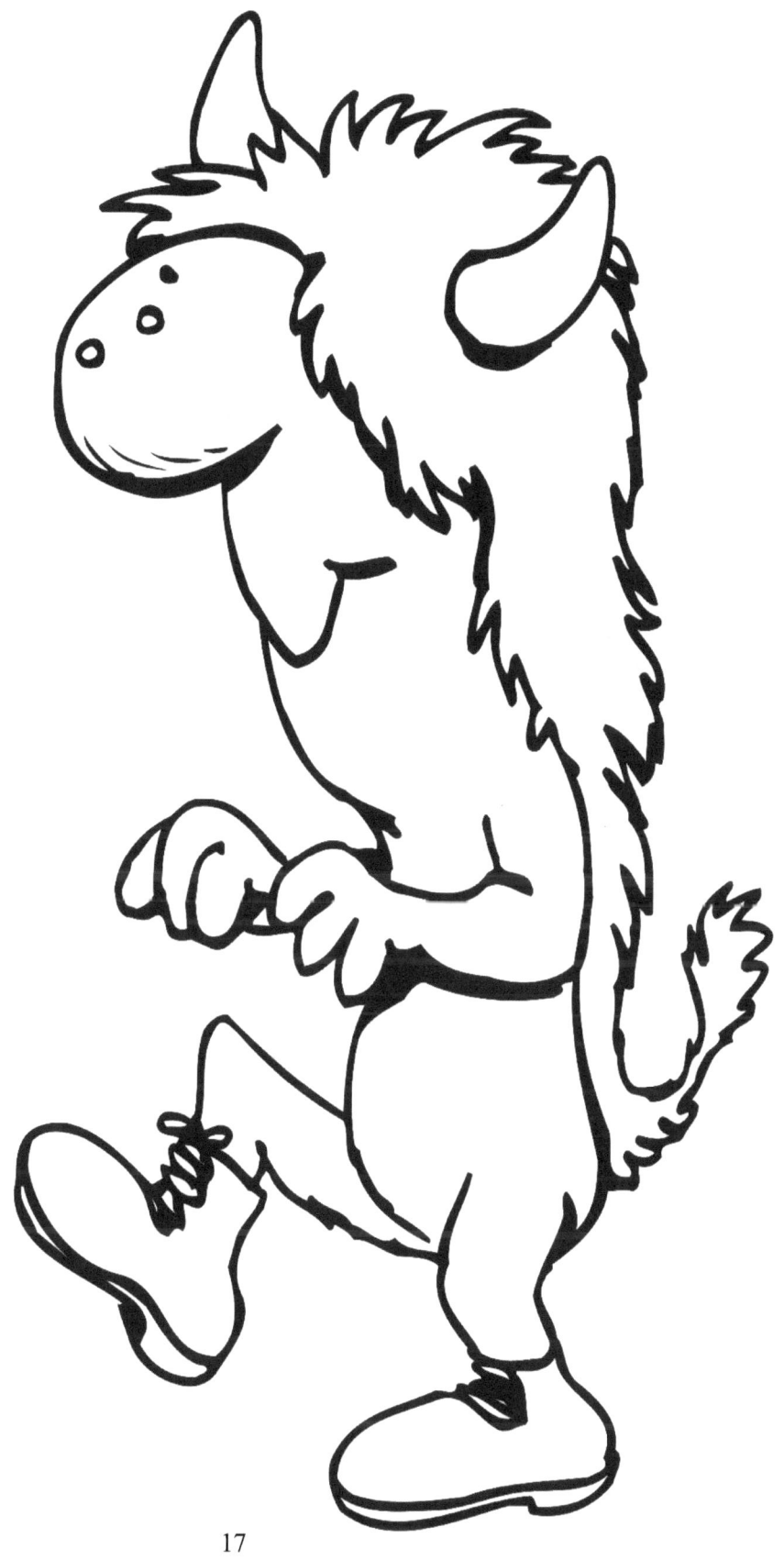

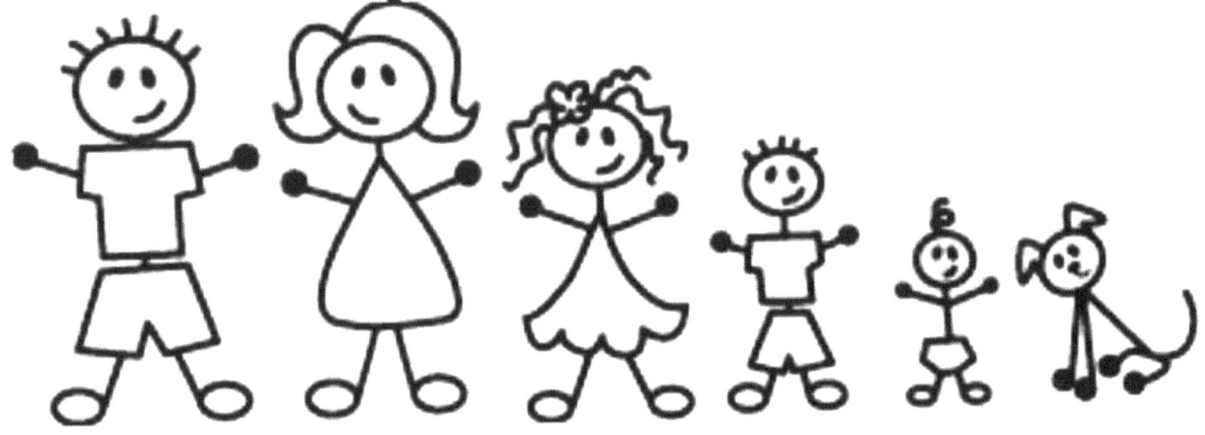

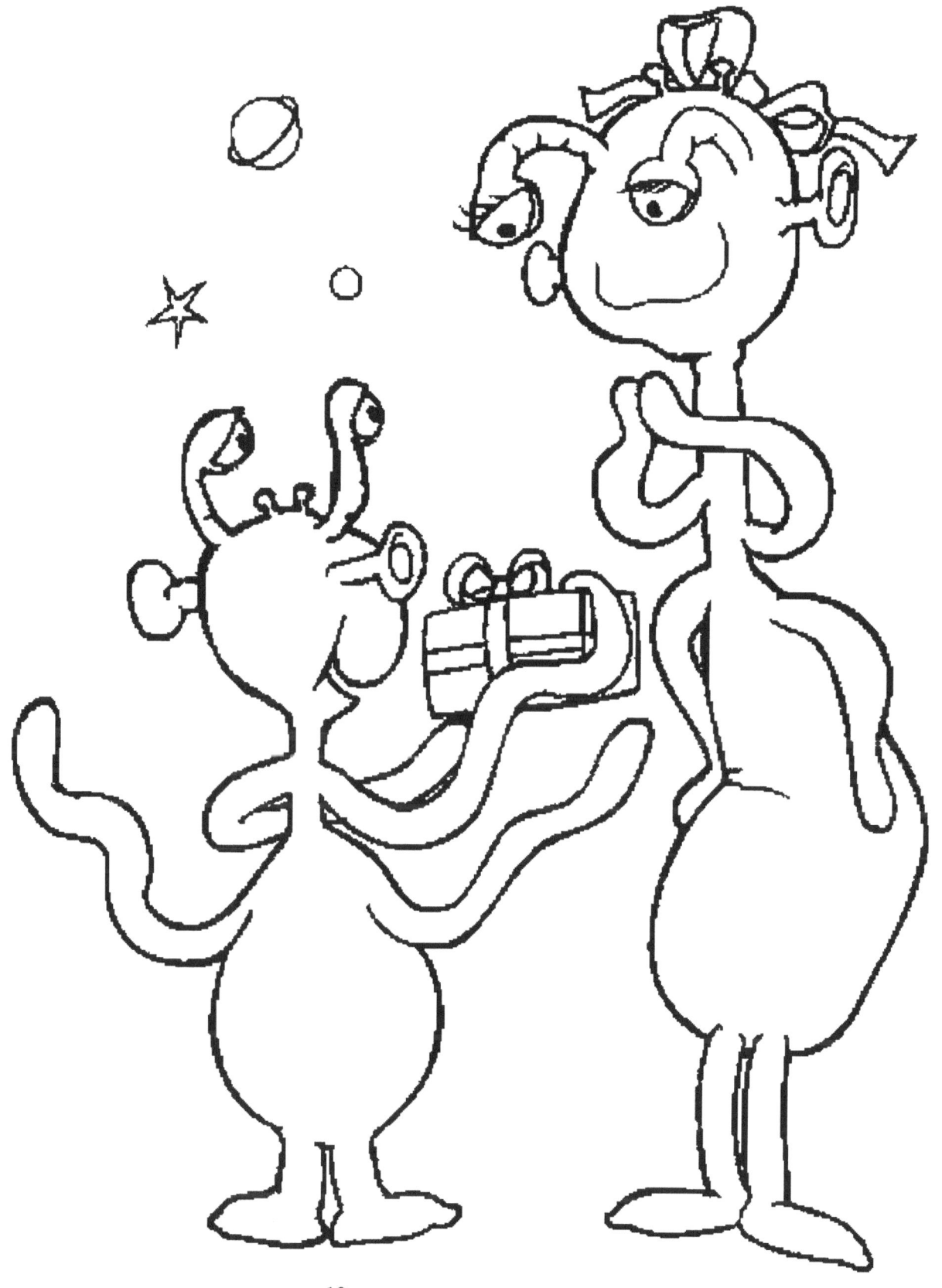

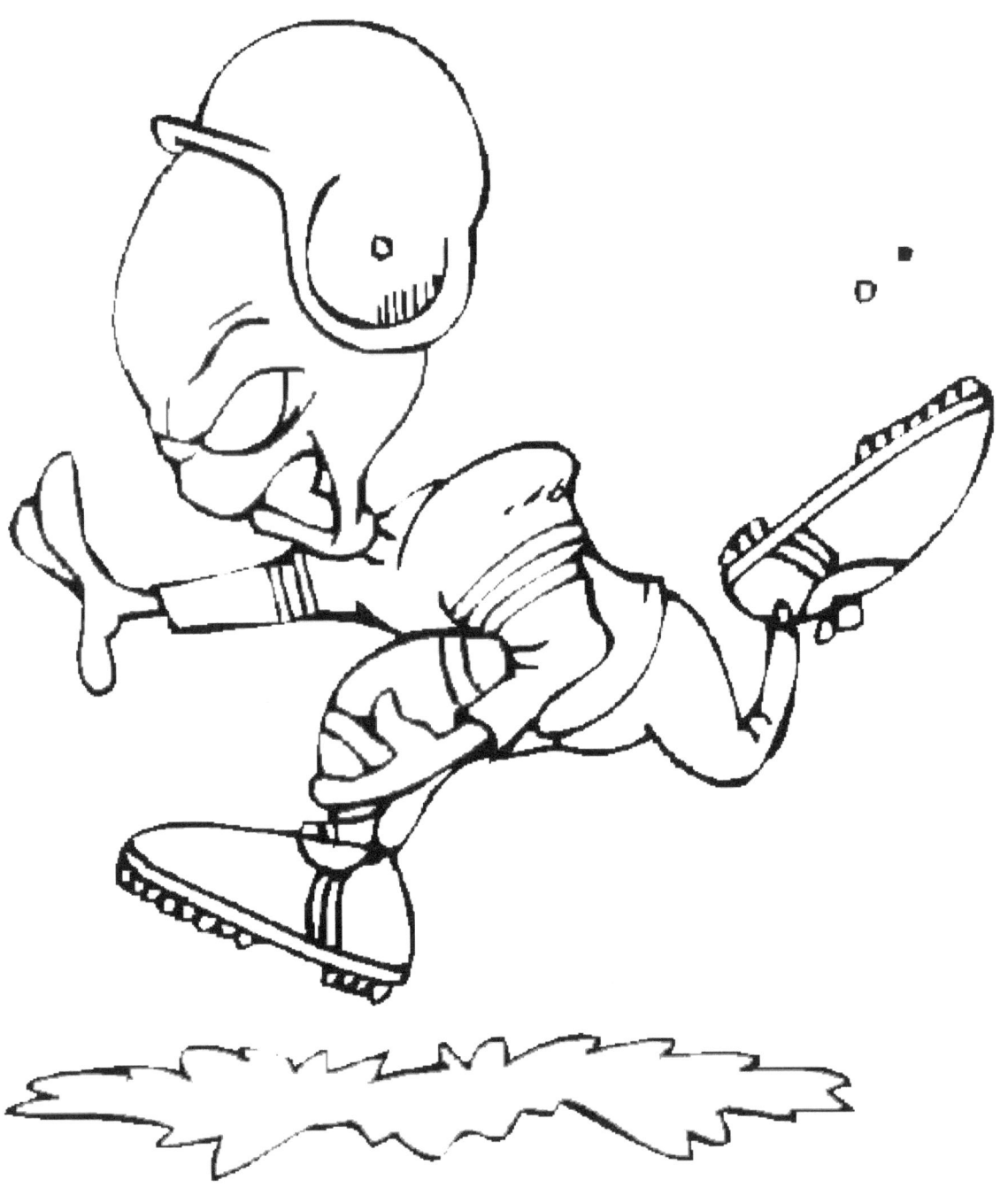

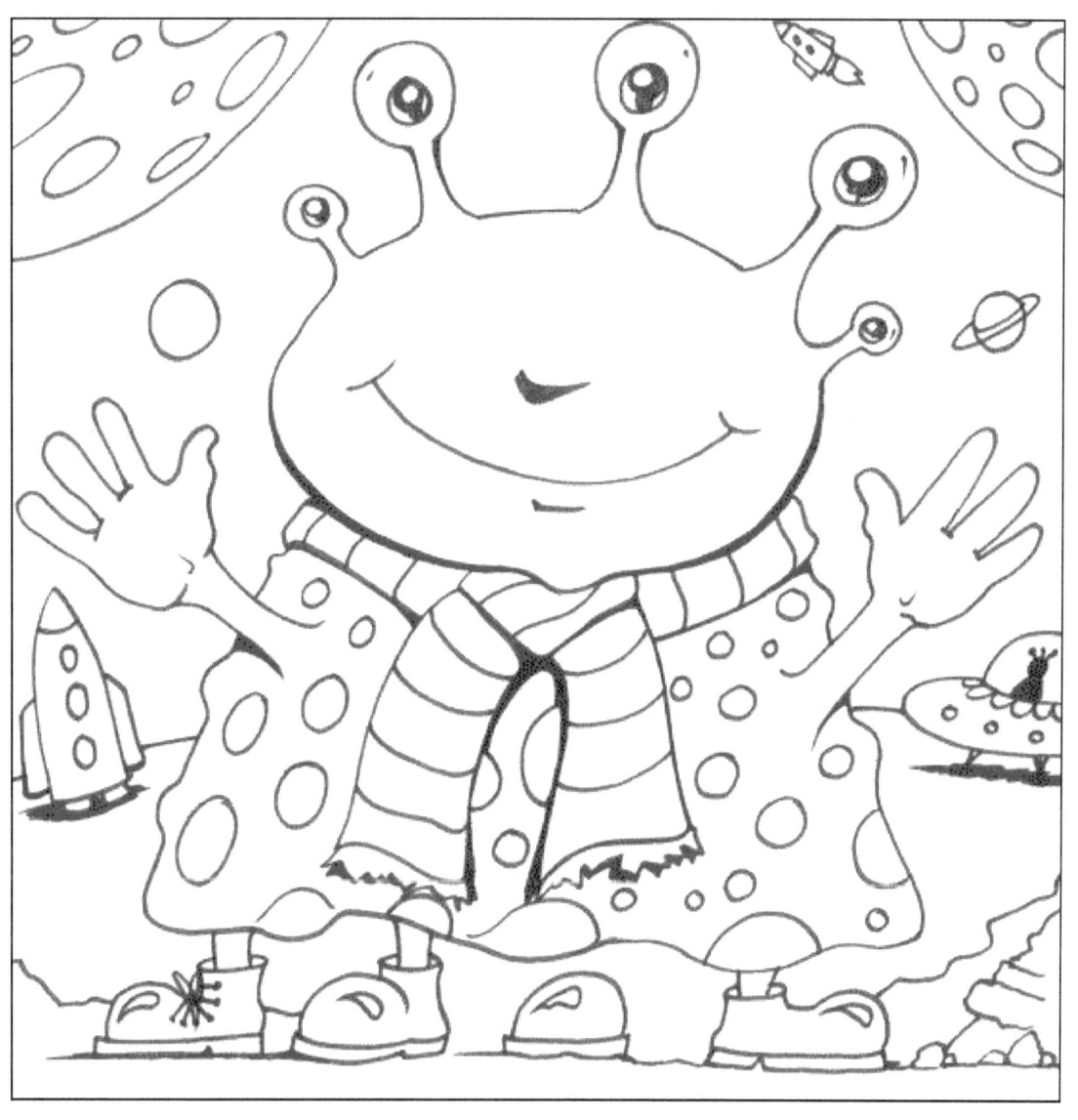

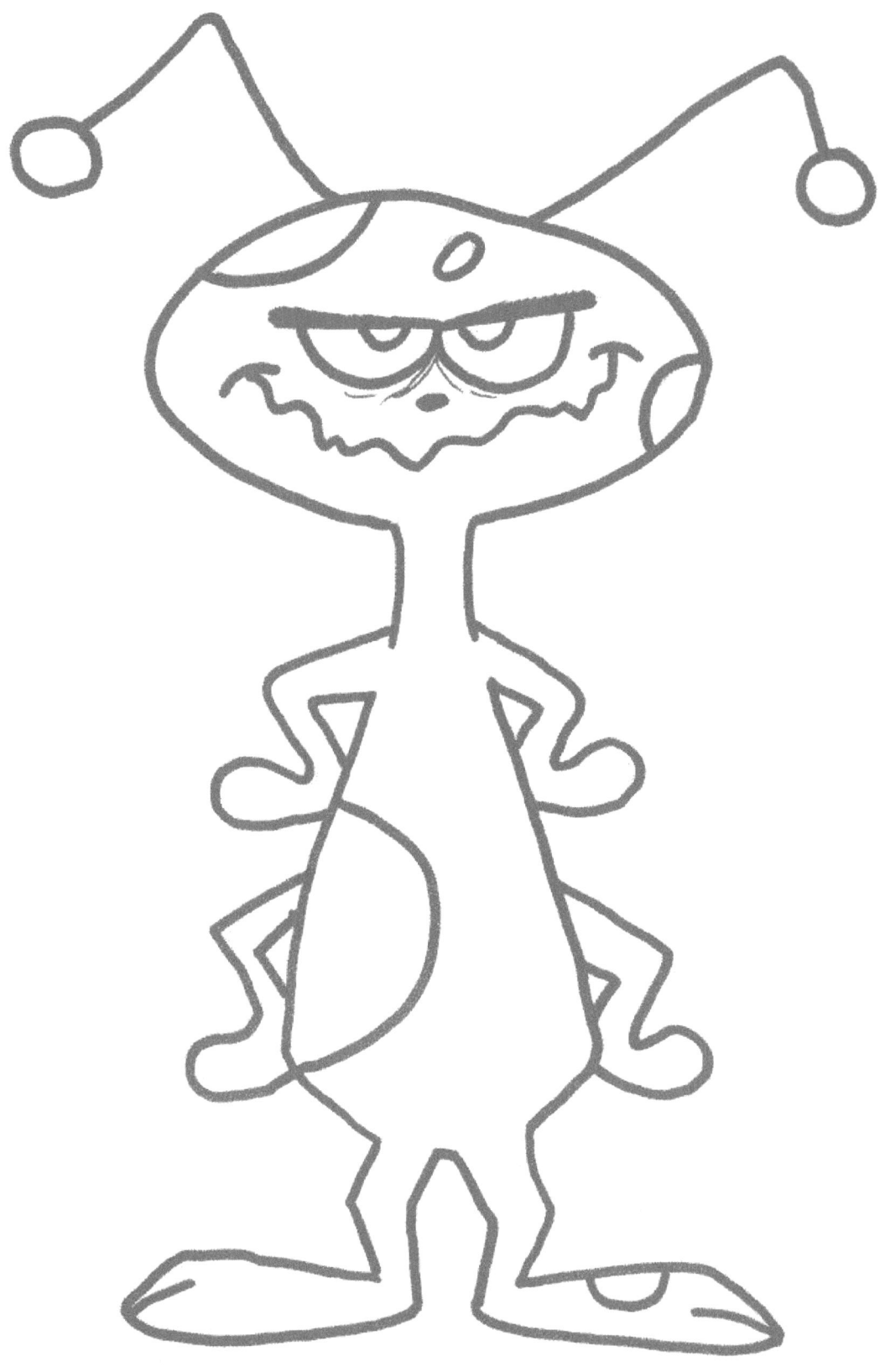

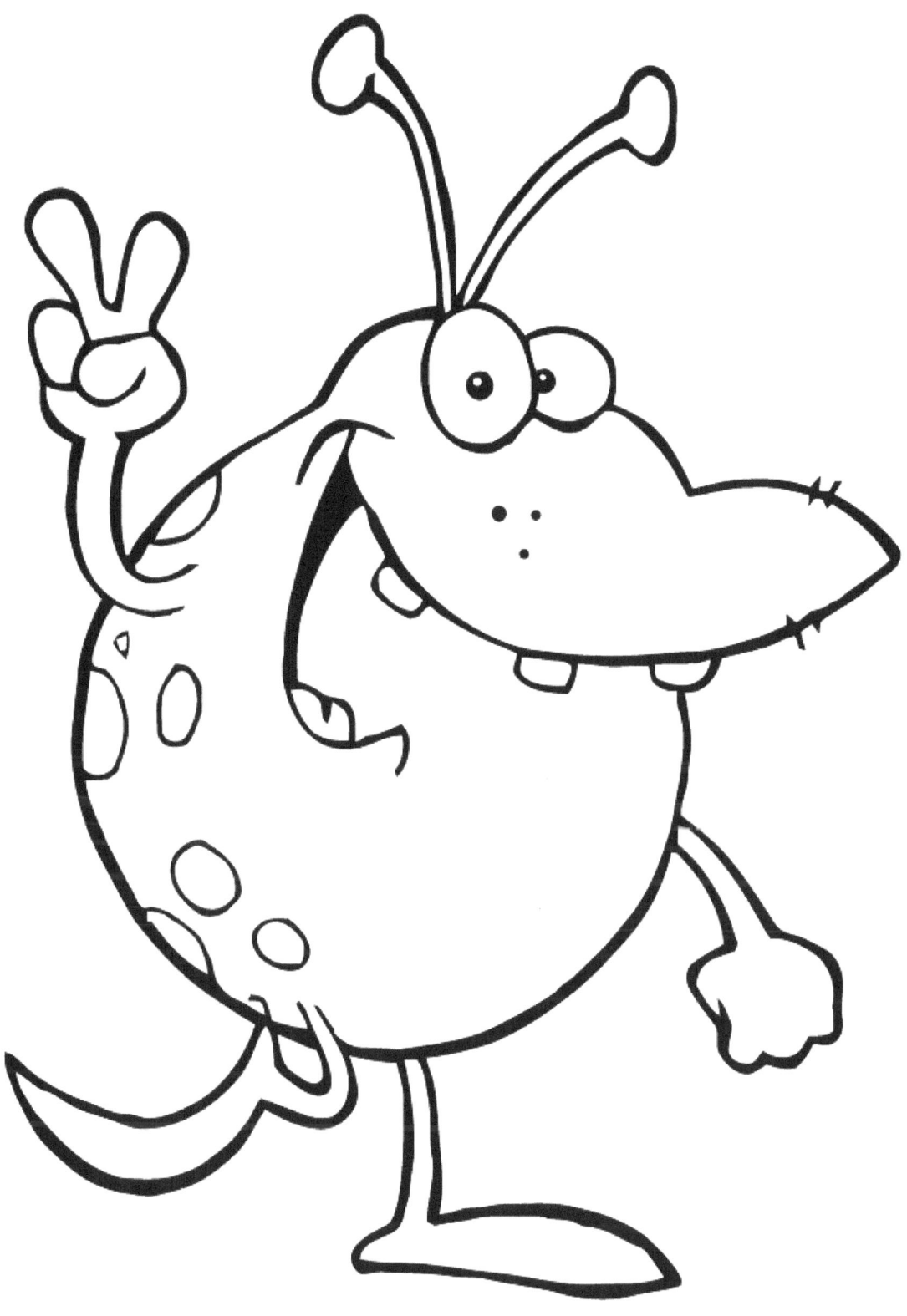

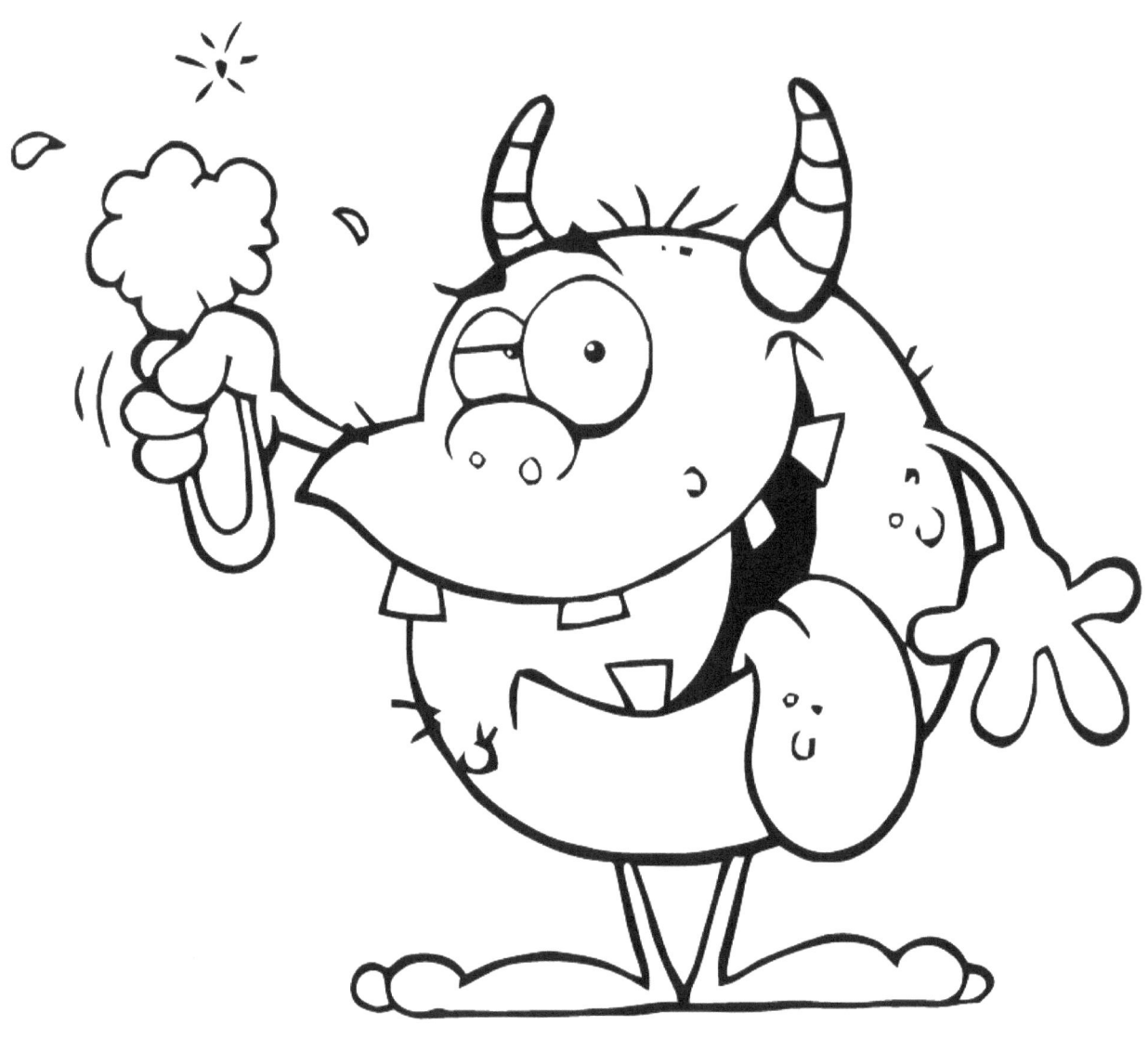

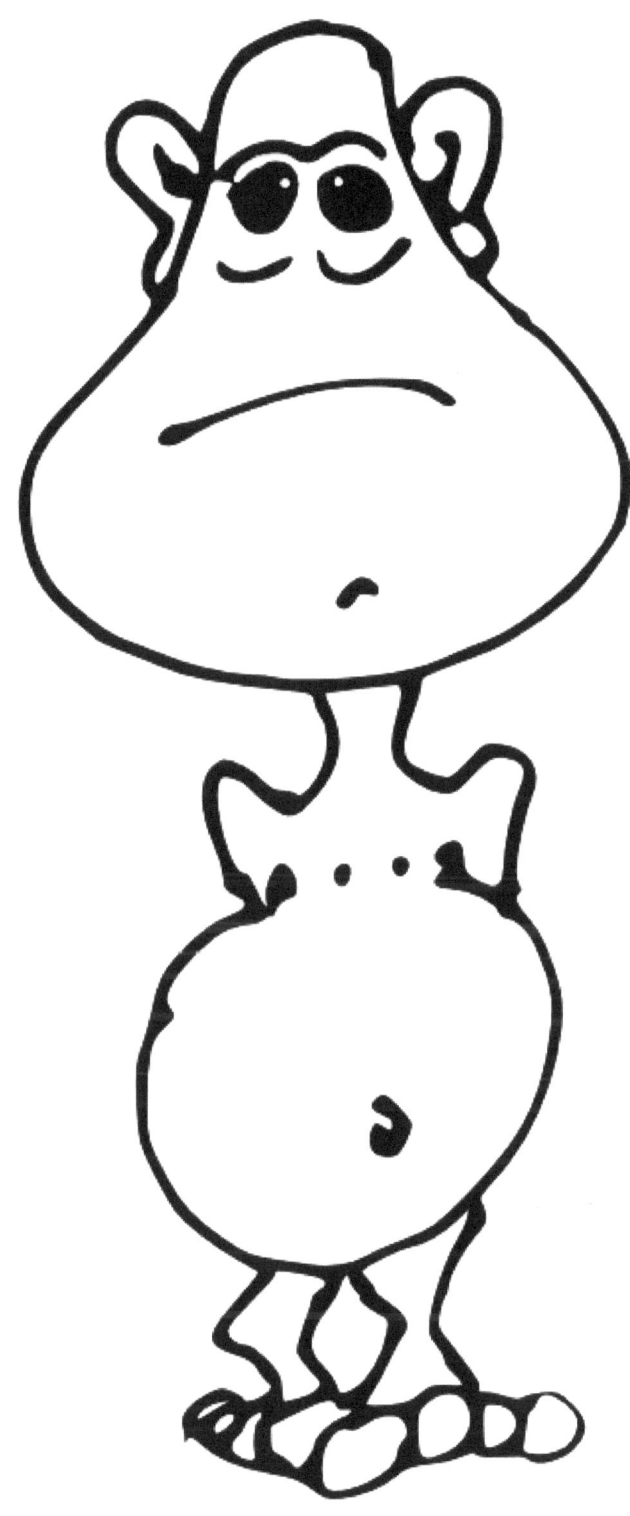

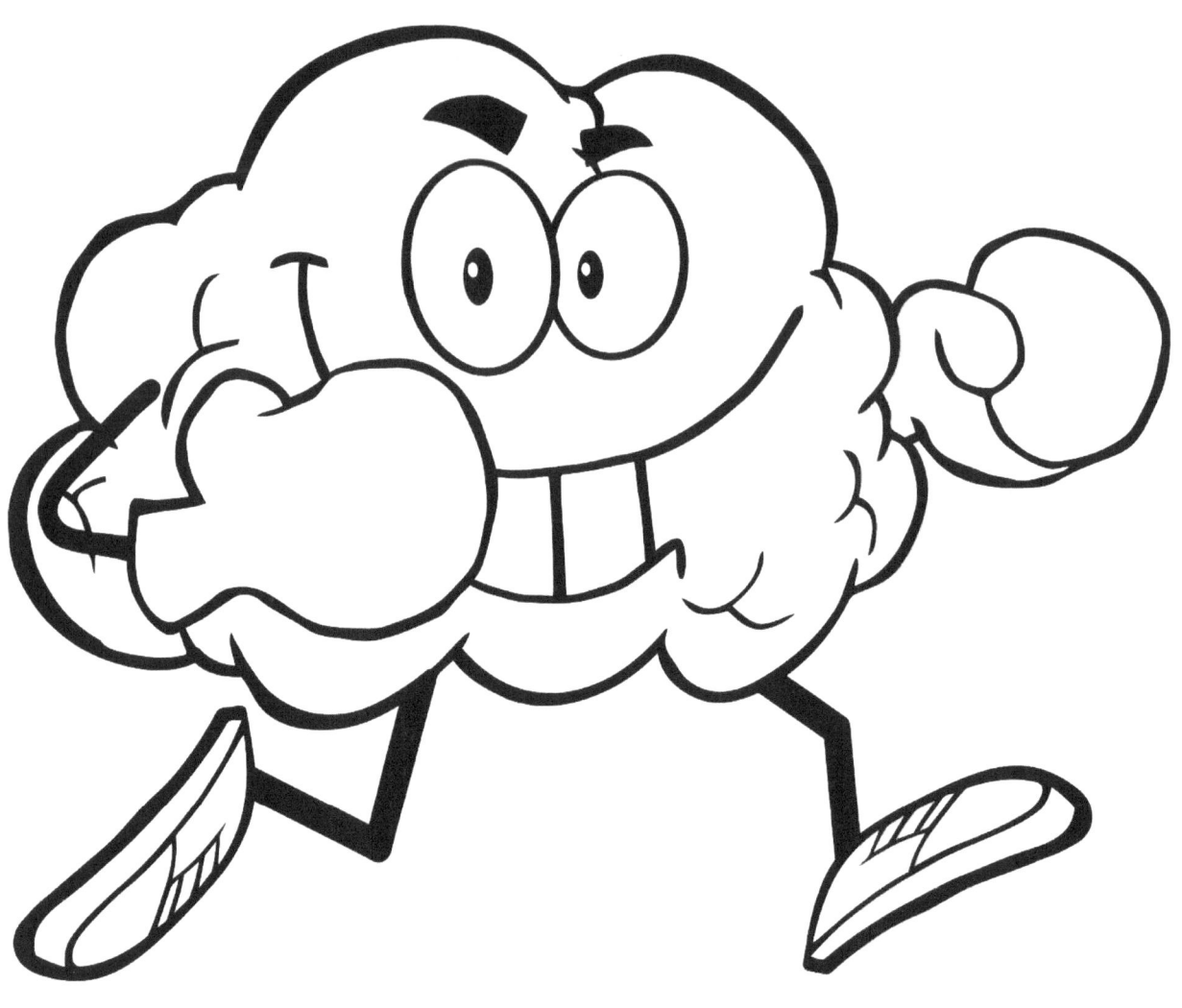

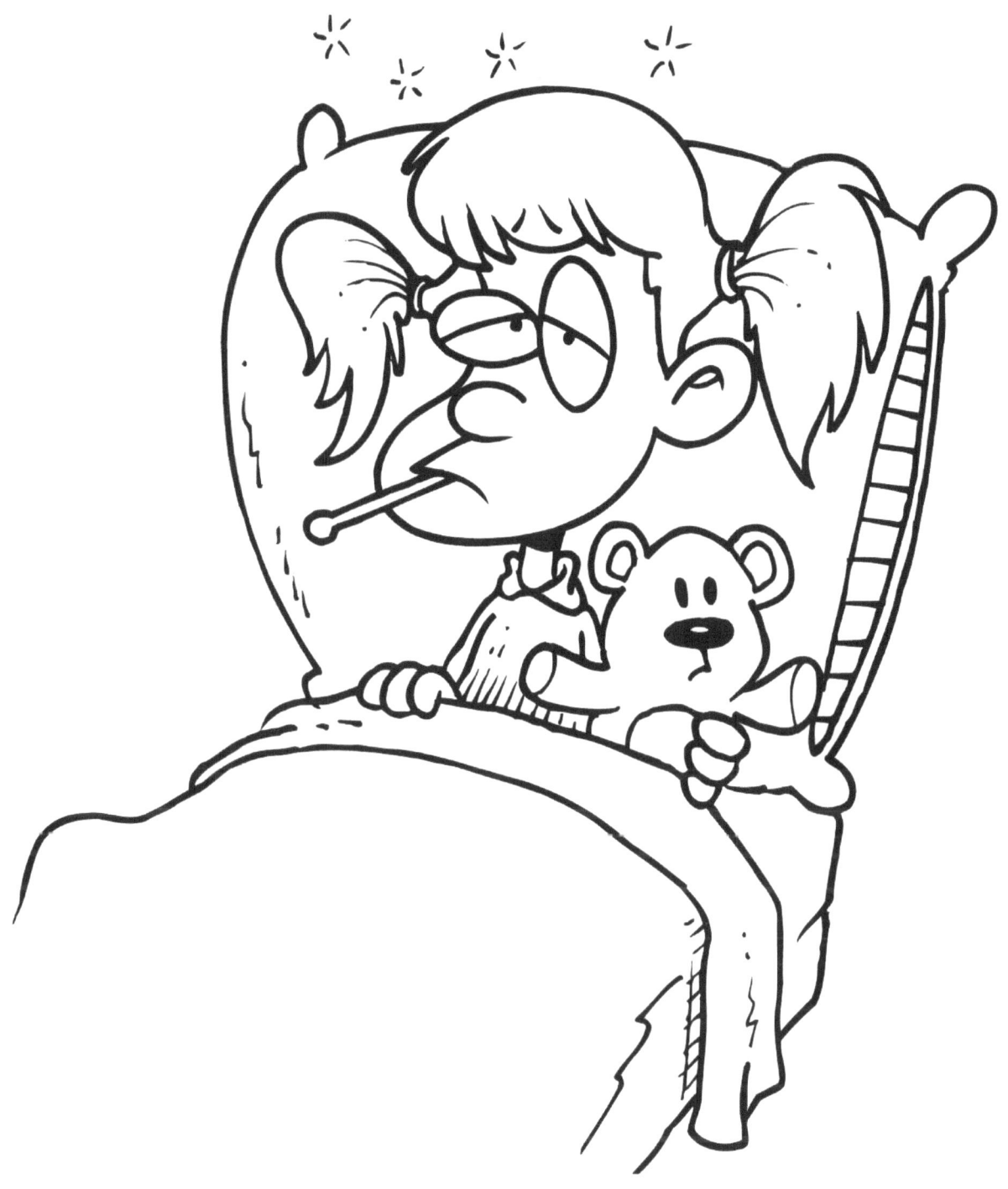

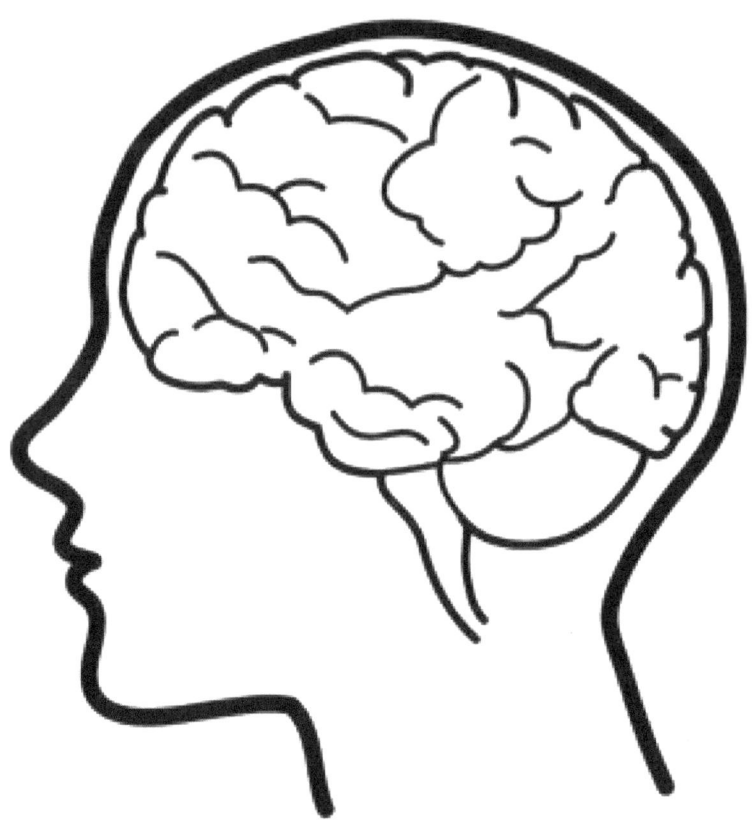

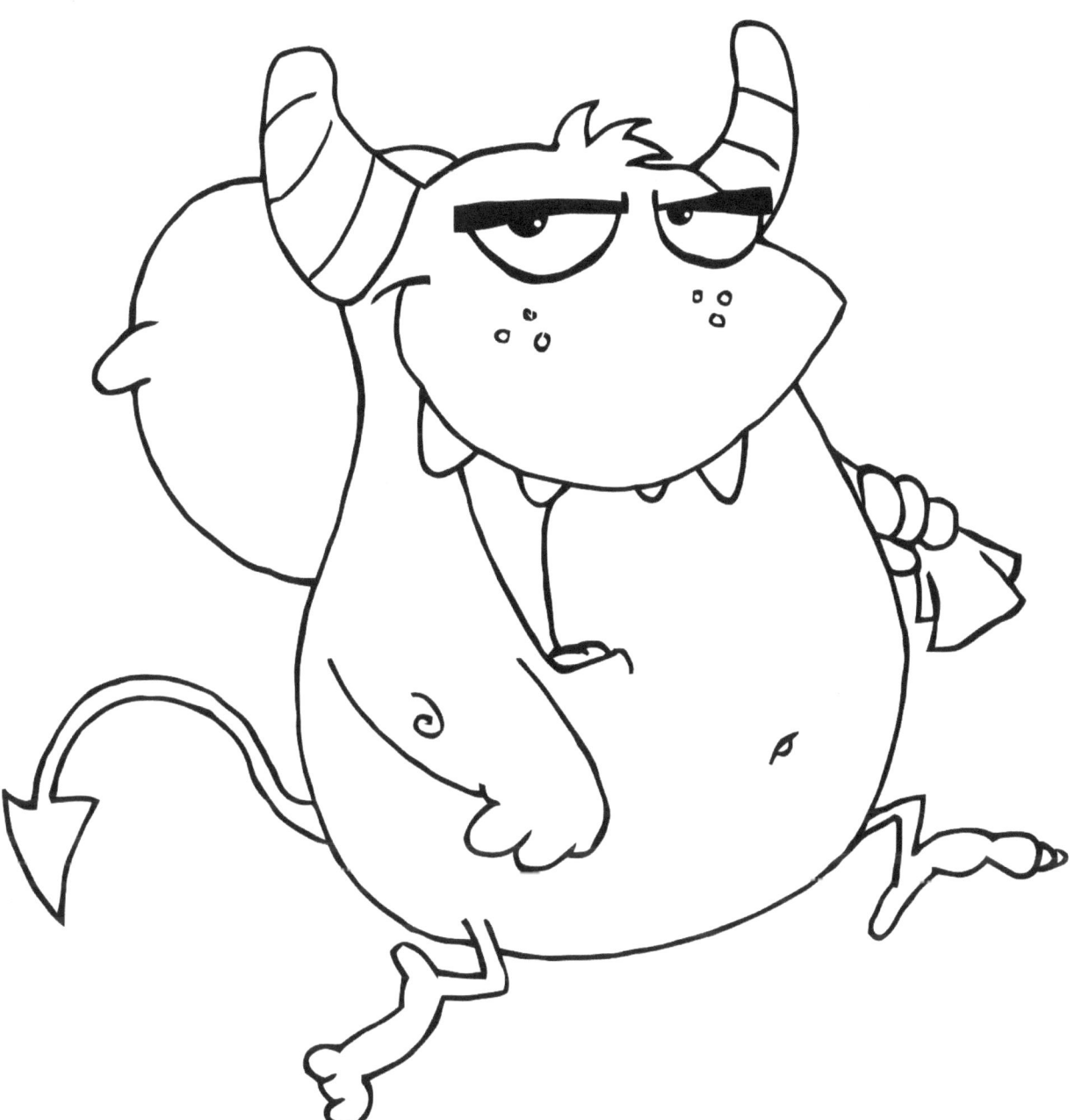

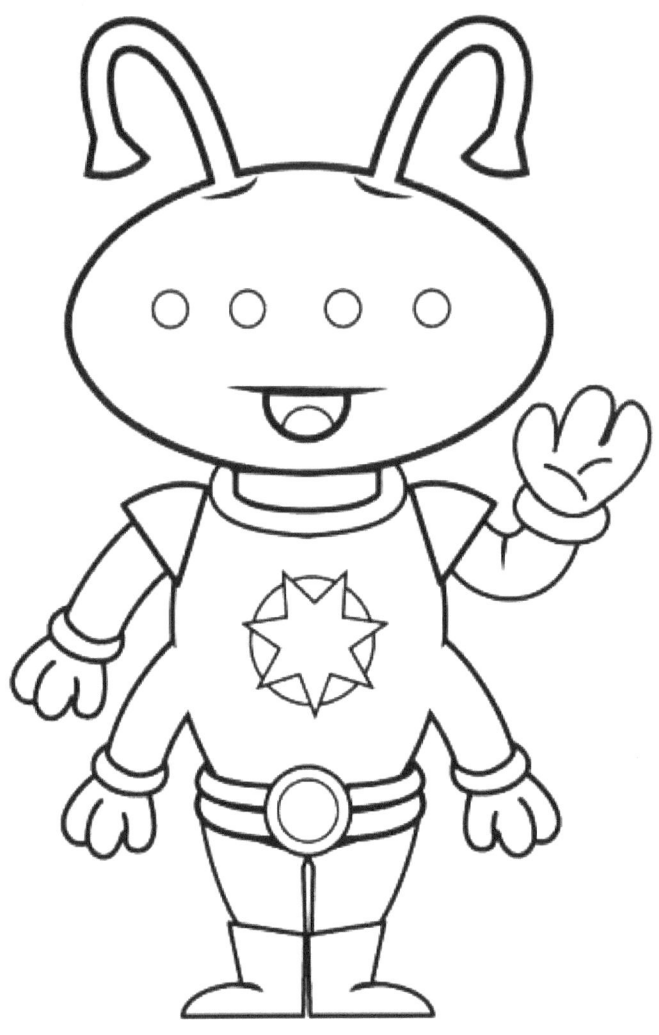

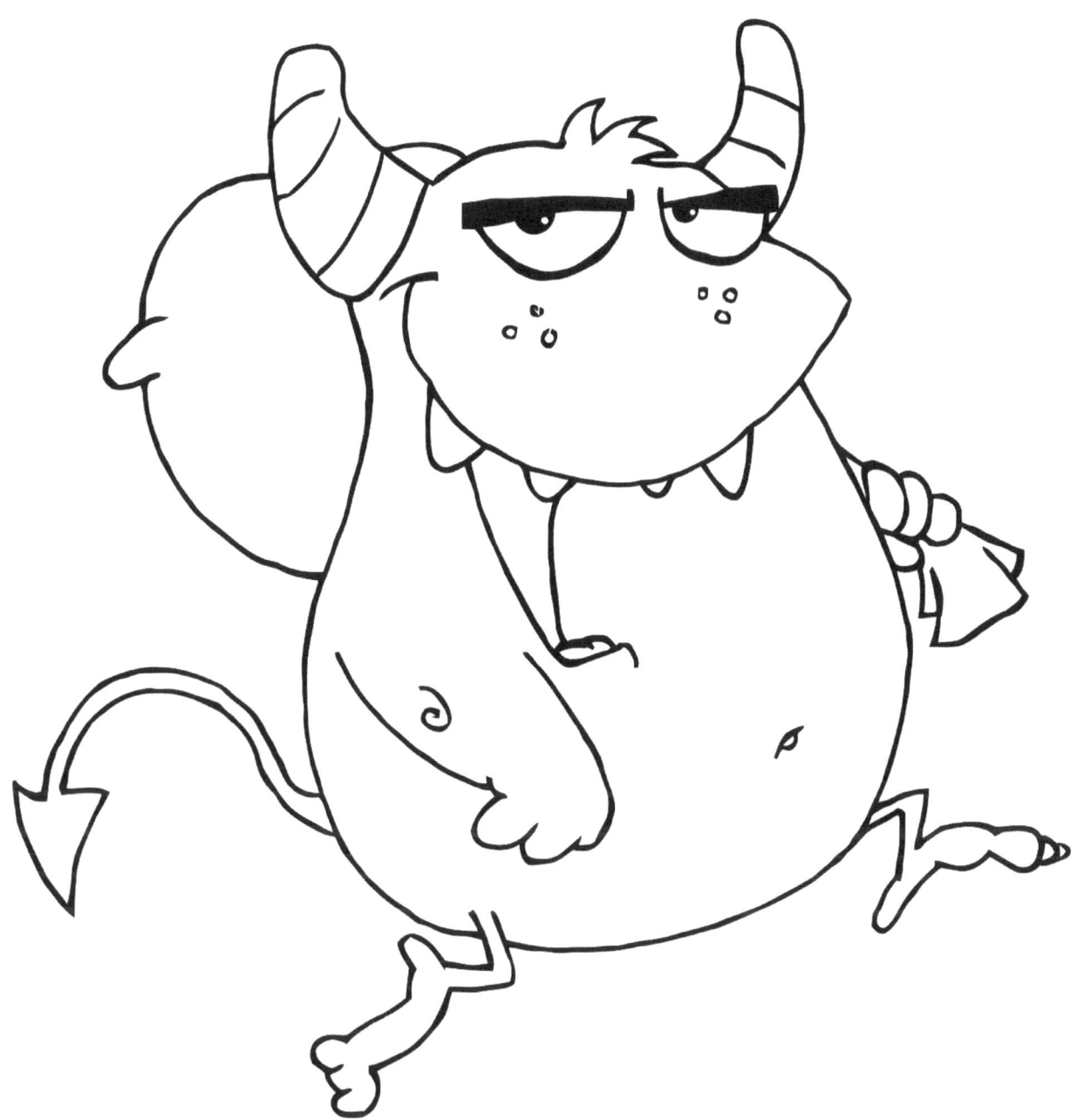

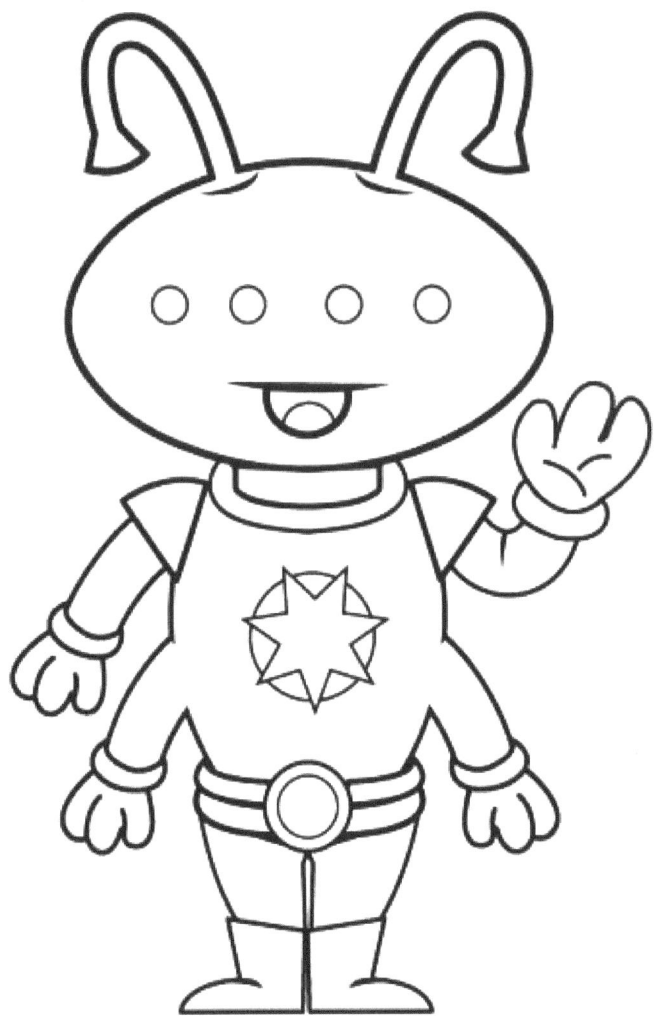

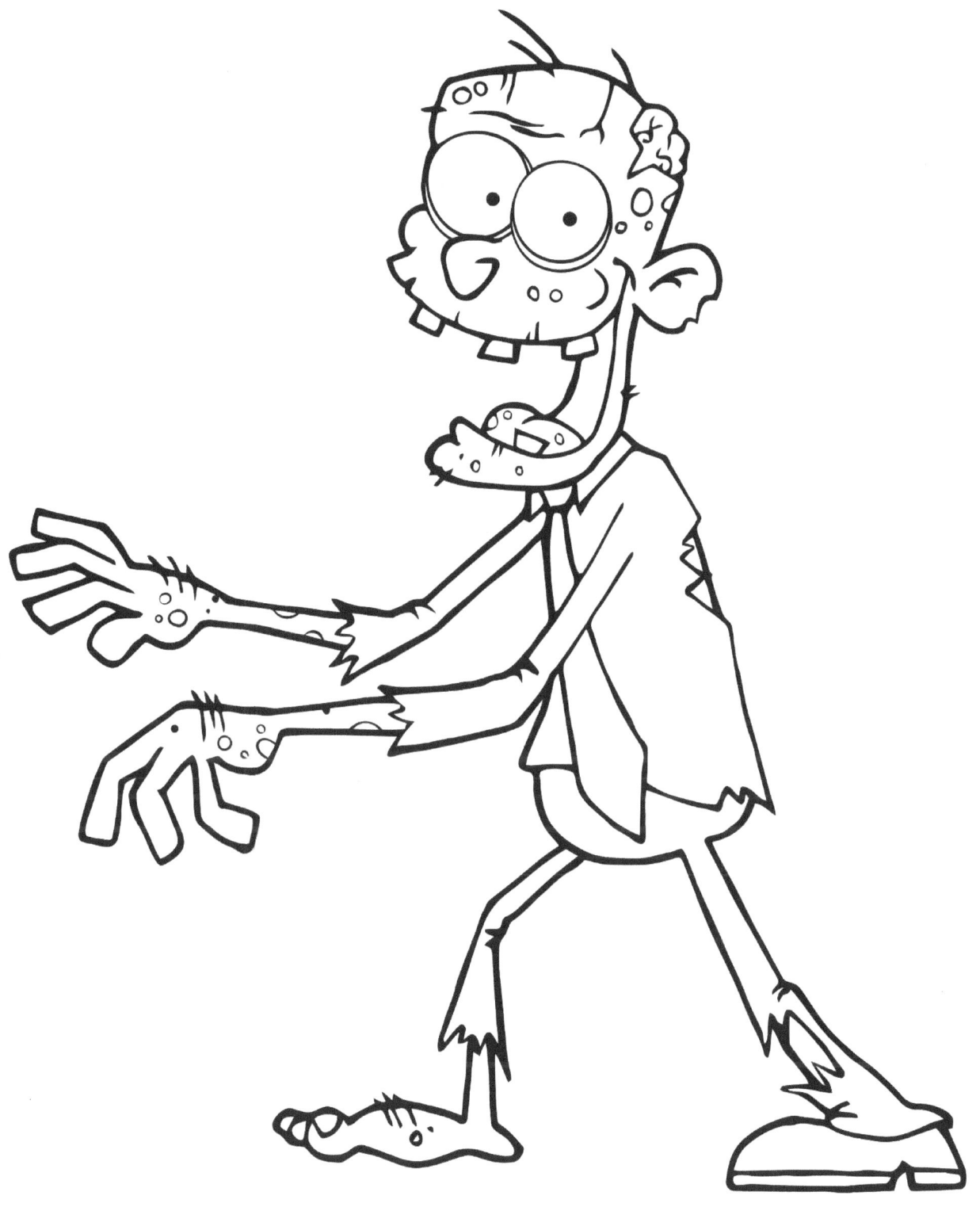

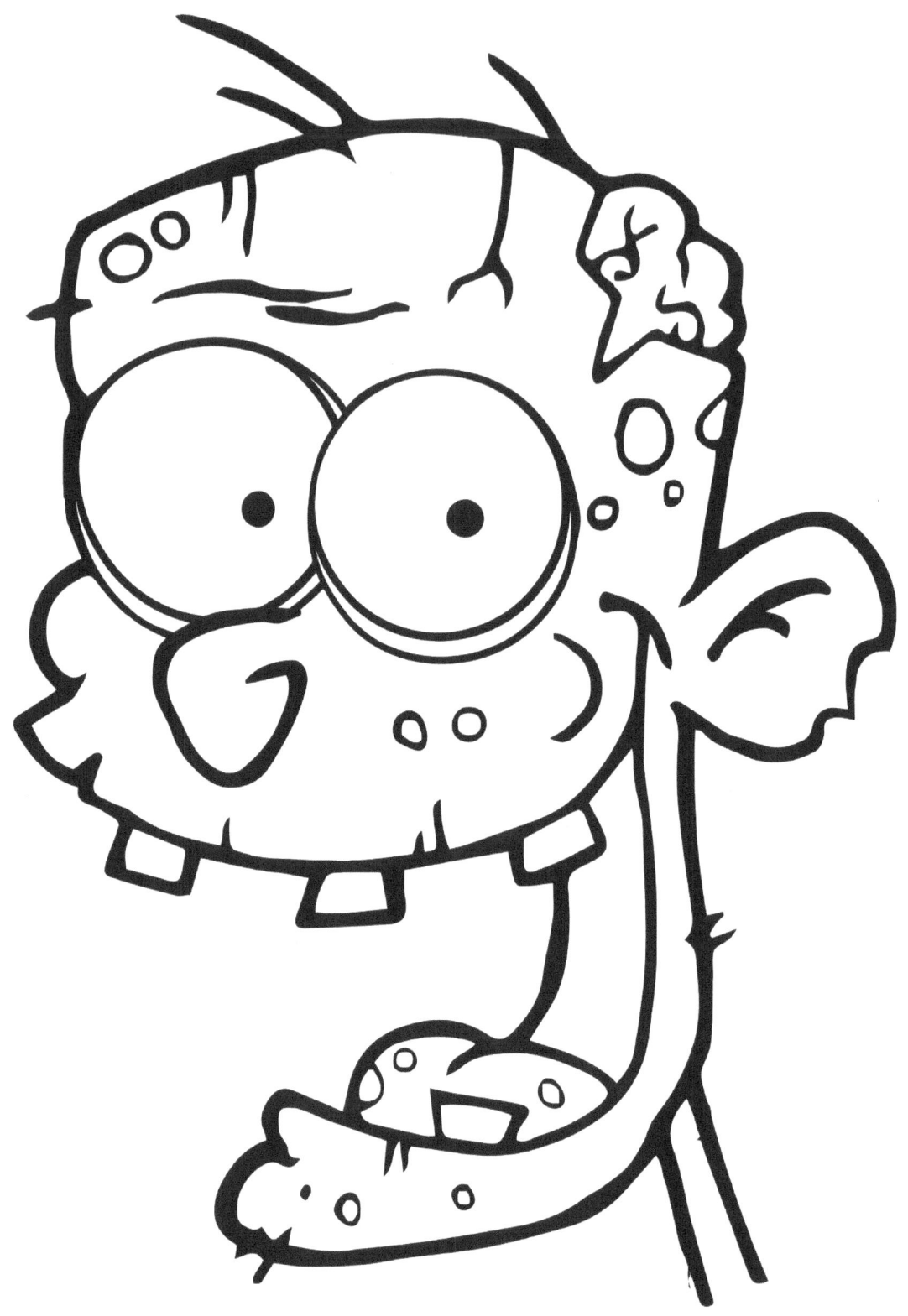

ABOUT THE AUTHOR

Renee Robinson's career began with publishing a series of poetry books while working on a biography about family, and life with cancer.

On of her most exciting accomplishments is the new Children Book Series, Holiday Adventures. Each child is welcome to visit lovable kittens Spooky and Boo as the learn about each holiday they experience for the first time. A Bonus chapter is added allowing the child extra interaction with the characters by getting to color them and some scenes from a book.

www.ingramcontent.com/pod-product-compliance
Lightning Source LLC
Chambersburg PA
CBHW050837180526
45159CB00004B/1932